SOCIAL NETWORK SITES FOR SCIENTISTS

CHANDOS
INFORMATION PROFESSIONAL SERIES

Series Editor: Ruth Rikowski
(email: Rikowskigr@aol.com)

Chandos' new series of books is aimed at the busy information professional. They have been specially commissioned to provide the reader with an authoritative view of current thinking. They are designed to provide easy-to-read and (most importantly) practical coverage of topics that are of interest to librarians and other information professionals. If you would like a full listing of current and forthcoming titles, please visit www.chandospublishing.com.

New authors: we are always pleased to receive ideas for new titles; if you would like to write a book for Chandos, please contact Dr Glyn Jones on g.jones.2@elsevier.com or telephone +44 (0) 1865 843000.

SOCIAL NETWORK SITES FOR SCIENTISTS

A QUANTITATIVE SURVEY

JOSÉ LUIS ORTEGA

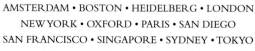

AMSTERDAM • BOSTON • HEIDELBERG • LONDON
NEW YORK • OXFORD • PARIS • SAN DIEGO
SAN FRANCISCO • SINGAPORE • SYDNEY • TOKYO
Chandos Publishing is an imprint of Elsevier

ELSEVIER

CP
CHANDOS
PUBLISHING

Chandos Publishing is an imprint of Elsevier
50 Hampshire Street, 5th Floor, Cambridge, MA 02139, United States
The Boulevard, Langford Lane, Kidlington, OX5 1GB, United Kingdom

Notices
Knowledge and best practice in this field are constantly changing. As new research and
experience broaden our understanding, changes in research methods, professional practices, or
medical treatment may become necessary.

Practitioners and researchers must always rely on their own experience and knowledge in
evaluating and using any information, methods, compounds, or experiments described herein. In
using such information or methods they should be mindful of their own safety and the safety of
others, including parties for whom they have a professional responsibility.

To the fullest extent of the law, neither the Publisher nor the authors, contributors, or editors,
assume any liability for any injury and/or damage to persons or property as a matter of products
liability, negligence or otherwise, or from any use or operation of any methods, products,
instructions, or ideas contained in the material herein.

British Library Cataloguing-in-Publication Data
A catalogue record for this book is available from the British Library

Library of Congress Cataloging-in-Publication Data
A catalog record for this book is available from the Library of Congress

ISBN: 978-0-08-100592-7 (Print)
ISBN: 978-0-08-100589-7 (Online)

For information on all Chandos Publishing
visit our website at https://www.elsevier.com/

  Working together
to grow libraries in
developing countries

www.elsevier.com • www.bookaid.org

Publisher: Glyn Jones
Acquisition Editor: Glyn Jones
Editorial Project Manager: Harriet Clayton
Production Project Manager: Debasish Ghosh
Designer: Mark Rogers

Typeset by MPS Limited, Chennai, India

To my mother, my father, my brothers and sister; to my friends, to everybody that believed that I would be able to do it . . . siempre nos quedará Torrox!

A tí, Kika, mi compañera fiel que tanto te sacrificas en hacer mis sueños realidad.

CONTENTS

LIST OF FIGURES

LIST OF TABLES

PREFACE

This tour among the social networking places for scientists has been an amazing voyage across an unexplored territory full of interesting revalations on the behaviour of the scholarly community in online collaborative environments. As an explorer scouting remote islands, through this survey I have been able to penetrate a complex world where academic relationships are projected and dissemination practices are reproduced. Thus, thanks to this exploration, it has been possible to detail what types of researchers are involved in these spaces, the way in which scholars are utilizing the functionalities of these services and what importance these spaces have for research activity and evaluation. This study has, for the first time, gathered together the most varied sample of social academic sites in order to represent the broad typology of services existing today addressed to making scientific contact. This has allowed me to extract precise information on their characteristics and functioning which has enabled specific indicators to be defined that facilitate easy comparison among them.

However, the most original and interesting aspect of this work is the employment of a quantitative approximation to the analysis of this world. Up to now, most of the studies faced with this reality have been focused on the opinion of scholars about the use of these platforms through a qualitative methodology (surveys, questionnaires, etc.). But this approach is limited to a small and subjective sample and only informs us of the tastes and preferences of the users. However, the quantitative approach brings an opportunity to complement this information, offering an objective view centred on the usage of these platforms and the behaviour of their users. But this systematic and quantitative approach can only can be carried out with the use of powerful crawlers and harvesters that extract and compile the information on each platform. This approach, originating in webometric studies, involves the extraction of huge volumes of information and the definition of indicators that permit the comparison and contextualization of each platform. From this point of view, this book presents novel and different results on the relationships of researchers with these platforms and the way in which these users collaborate among themselves.

The book begins with an introductory chapter in which social networking sites for scientists are put in the context of the Web 2.0 philosophy, the Open Access movement and the altmetrics phenomenon.

In addition, this chapter describes the methods and instruments used to accomplish this study. Next, in the first of the chapters on analysis the structure and functioning of Nature Network and BiomedExperts is described, the first services that attempted to develop a social platform for scholars. However, these disappeared and the pioneering spaces are analysed to show how these first attempts at social networking sites were born from different conceptions. The next chapter reviews CiteULike and BibSonomy, the most representative of the social bookmarking services that illustrate the impact of folksonomy and social tagging in the development of the first social networking spaces. The following chapter analyses Mendeley and Zotero to get into the world of reference management tools and the huge possibilities they contain for bibliographic search. This chapter discusses how these services fit into the social networking world. ResearchGate and Academia.edu, dissected in the next chapter, are the most important examples of document sharing sites. These platforms could be considered the last stage in the evolution of social networking sites, revealing document sharing as the main interactive activity among researchers. The penultimate chapter is a comparative exercise that benchmarks the performance of each site in relation to the others, as a way to point out differences across types of services and detect the success and failure of each platform. Finally, a concluding chapter comments on the main results of this study and discusses their implications for academic activity in the Web.

However, this project would never have got off the ground without the inestimable technical support of the Cybermetric Lab, which put at my disposal a full array of computers working day and night crawling and harvesting information from every platform studied. Without this strong technical support, this quantitative analysis never would never have seen the light of day. I would also like to thank Isidro Aguillo whose insightful reviews and comments led me to improve the results and enhance the conclusions.

ABOUT THE AUTHOR

José Luis Ortega is a web researcher from the Spanish National Research Council (CSIC). He achieved a fellowship in the Cybermetrics Lab of the CSIC where he finished his doctoral studies (2003–8). In 2005, he was hired by the Virtual Knowledge Studio of the Royal Netherlands Academy of Sciences and Arts and in 2008 was offfered a full position in the CSIC as an information scientist. Now, he continues to collaborate with the Cybermetrics Lab in research areas such as webometrics, web usage mining, visualization of information, social network analysis, web bibliometrics, etc.

CHAPTER 1

Introduction

1.1 THE WEB AND THE WEB 2.0 CONCEPT

At the dawn of the new century the Web had become consolidated into all aspects of life, this new and revolutionary information technology has transformed the information habits of the entire world and had made possible the immediate diffusion of content to any part of the globe. Born into the academic environment, the Net soon reached every facet of human activity, turning information into an important transformational asset for the rising knowledge society (Castells, 2010). The successful changes brought about by this disruptive technology do not simply rely on instant access to an enormous amount of data, videos, pictures, etc., but on the possibility of avoiding those mediators that, at that time, controlled the information flows. This singular characteristic meant that users would became publishers and distributors of their own creations, without any gatekeeper to censure or take advantage of its position (Van Dijck, 2009). Authors that published their own books online, little shops that offered their products direct to the consumer and businesses that advertised themselves on fancy web pages proliferated exponentially. Thus a great part of the information that ran through the Web was content created by its own users, being at the same time sources and receivers according to communication theory (Morris & Ogan, 1996).

In spite of this revolutionary change in the communication process, this world remained linear, unidirectional and static, where users only surfed the Web to look for information or built fixed websites (Cormode & Krishnamurthy, 2008). However, several technological advances led to the development of a more dynamic environment at the start of the twenty-first century. New protocols (SOAP), languages (XML, RDF) and formats (RSS) were developed by the industry to facilitate the expansion of electronic commerce on the Web. This sector demanded spaces online where commercial transactions were easy, fast and safe. In this way the Web was converted into a platform for services from where users could now not only search for information, but carry out any type of action (Jarvenpaa & Todd, 1996). Now, we have changed from searching for

Social Network Sites for Scientists.
ISBN 978-0-08-100592-7

flights to buying the ticket, from knowing the requirements for a service to directly applying for that service and from visiting a friend's homepage to looking at the postings on their wall.

The concept of Web 2.0 emerged to describe the great changes that these new solutions were already bringing about on the Web (Knorr, 2003; O'Reilly, 2007). The concept pointed out that these alterations were not just improvements and upgrades but were going to modify the way in which users interacted with the Web and, even more, the way in which society itself was being transformed by the Web. Under this new transactional environment, the Web also started to produce new spaces where users could participate in the production of content. If users can already buy goods online or file paperwork with the government, now they can exchange and manage content with other partners as well. Wikipedia (2001) could be considered the first collaborative enterprise that attempted to create a universal encyclopaedia with entries written by anyone and on any issue in the world. Its model flawlessly represented the spirit of Web 2.0, the creation of a self-managed information system in which the contents are created by an online community of altruistic members. The success of Wikipedia, with more than 5 million entries today[1] demonstrated that collaborative actions could achieve great purposes without the supervised oversight of publishers, distributors, content companies, etc. This collaborative effort was extended and new applications were derived from the same paradigm. Delicious (2003), perhaps the best example of the new Web 2.0, was created as a service to label or tag viewed content on the Web. As a kind of bookmark page, this platform allowed the creation and management of personal libraries of favourite web resources. Although functionally this had already been implemented by all the web browsers, the great contribution of this platform was the utilization of two key elements that would define the upcoming social services on the Web. Firstly, these personal collections of references could be shared with other members, thus allowing these posts to be reused by the online community, which could edit, correct and comment on these same items again. The second innovation was that those references were organized using keywords or tags that each user freely added, creating an interconnected system of categories that structured these contents. This networking behaviour generated a global knowledge system in which the information would be produced and categorized using the collaborative will of the people. In the same way, hundreds of sites emerged applying this philosophy to any type of materials. Social platforms for sharing videos (YouTube, Vimeo), photographs (Flickr, Instagram), music (Last.fm), news (Digg, Reddit, Slashdot), messages (Twitter, Tumblr) and documents (Scribd, SlideShare) appeared everywhere extending this model to any facet of life. This indexing method was not exclusive to social networking sites but was spreading to other information systems such as directories and search engines. The most interesting thing is that this model shaped a new social awareness of the importance of the community in the production of content and the power of the group to filter and select valuable information. All these platforms demonstrated that there was an important community of web users interested in collaborative projects and had evidence that social networking would produce successful and profitable products.

1.2 SOCIAL NETWORKING SITES – THE WEB OF THE PEOPLE

In this context, platforms were created whose only purpose was to put users in touch with other users. The first social networking sites, Friendster (2002) and MySpace (2003), functioned as personal directories where their members could meet other friends through the network of acquaintances. However, the first genuine web service that would change the concept of online social networks was Facebook (2004). Born as a restricted network for American scholars, its spread worldwide did not commence until the restrictions to signing up were removed in 2006. Five years later, it became the largest social platform with around 1 billion users (Ostrow, 2011). Its success fundamentally rested on the fact that their profiles were not just members' calling cards but that they constituted a real space where users could express themselves posting texts, pictures, videos, etc. To some extent, these personal pages could be a kind of personal diary open only to a specific network of intimates that contained, in a multimedia form, all the main events in the lives of their users. This scheme, in which the content production was fundamental for establishing contacts, was disseminated and new specialized spaces, addressed to a specific public, were born. Vertical social networks (Lieb, 2013) now constitute the next challenge for online social network analysis and new specific services for small businesses (Wave), professionals (LinkedIn), programmers (GitHub), engineers (Spiceworks) and physicians (Doximity) are springing up everywhere.

But what is a social networking site (SNS)? Boyd and Ellison (2007) define 'social network sites as web-based services that allow individuals to (1) construct a public or semi-public profile within a bounded system, (2) articulate a list of other users with whom they share a connection, and (3) view and traverse their list of connections and those made by others within the system', considering that 'the public display of connections is a crucial component of SNSs'. However, although these elements, I think, could constitute an online social site by themselves, they are not sufficient to be a successful site. As can be seen in the above examples, it is fundamental that these social platforms incorporate instruments for producing and as well as adding content. In this sense, a social networking site could be defined as an online environment where users, besides creating personal profiles and establishing contact among themselves, they can also produce and insert content at disposal of their contacts or the entire community (Ellison & Boyd, 2013). This definition attempts to emphasise the informational aspect because the networking relationships might be just a consequence of the information flowing within the network. In other words, as more documents, images, videos, etc., are hosted on the system, more networking activity will be generated. In this way, an online space only can evolve if their members are able to produce, add and share information units among themselves. Hence content is the fuel of social networking.

1.3 OPEN ACCESS – TOWARD A NEW SCIENTIFIC COMMUNICATION

Before the concept of Web 2.0 was born and social networking sites made an appearance, one of the most critical movements almost since the start of the Web arose in the academic community. A long time ago, the academic publishing system had fallen into a severe crisis (Panitch & Michalak, 2005). The number of academic publications did nothing but increase, while subscription costs grew at a dramatic pace, far above inflation. This increase did not correspond with any significant reduction in the production costs of printing. In addition to this situation, throughout the past century a process of amalgamation among publishers along with rapid acquisition programmes for new journals caused the concentration of the system in the hands of just a few large publishing companies (Elsevier, Springer, Wiley, etc.). Those most affected in this system were the academic libraries which looked on as more and more of their budgets were allocated to the payment of subscriptions, resulting in a clear reduction of precious scientific funds to the benefit of large private corporations. This situation came to a head in 1997 when the Association of Research Libraries developed the Scholarly Publishing and Academic Resources Coalition (SPARC) and put forth a set of demands from scholarly libraries and other organizations in order to solve this critical situation and offer alternatives that could ease fair access to the scientific literature. But the scholarly community was already aware on these problems. Three years before, Stevan Harnad (1994) had launched his well-known 'Subversive Proposal', where he encouraged the free and open exchange of scientific literature, depositing copies of research articles in public academic servers accessible through the FTP protocol. Harnad's proposal was not ground-breaking by his own admission – the practice was already common in computing environments – but made explicit the existence of an alternative channel by which research results could be spread apart from the traditional publishing system. Thus the Web was able to emerge as an alternative way of avoiding the established publishing system, reducing costs, shortening publishing times and reaching wider audiences. In this case, the Web favoured the elimination of mediators as well, allowing direct communication between researchers without any limitation or fee.

Two main channels were established to make effective open access to the scholarly papers. The first channel were the electronic journals (gold open access) that duplicated the traditional model but were now without subscription and offered a reduced publication delay (Odlyzko, 1997). The *Bryn Mawr Classical Review* (1990), *Postmodern Culture* (1990) and *Psycoloquy* (1990) are a few examples of the first electronic journals that sprang up around the Web. However, this model was not compulsory and now most of the journals have an electronic version accessible through the major payment platforms owned by the academic publishing giants (ScienceDirect, IngentaConnect, Wiley Online, etc.). The second channel (green open access) was rather different and with a better fate. It consisted of the deposit of a full text copy of the manuscript in an open repository or digital archive before the paper was edited and published by the journal (Guédon, 2004; Harnad et al., 2004). This process avoids the slow publication times and assures the peer review of journals as well as the upcoming citation count. This protocol produced the flowering of thematic repositories such as ArXiv.org (1991) specializing in physics, the great biomedical deposit Pubmed (1997) and RePEc (1997) for the archiving of economics papers. Soon, it was common to upload pre-print copies of articles to a repository before being accepted for publication in a print journal. On the other hand, institutional repositories such as CERN Document

Server, the eScholarship Repository of the University of California and HAL (Hyper Articles en Ligne) are used to express the scientific power of an institution as well as demonstrating the commitment of their organizations to the transparency and democratization of science. Thanks to the Budapest Open Access Initiative (2012), a manifesto that defines the objectives of Open Access, these deposits were becoming institutionalized and achieved policy mandates that oblige the hosting of publicly funded results in open repositories – for instead, Horizon 2020 of the European Union (European Commission, 2013), the NIH Public Access Policy or the Research Councils UK (2013).

1.4 ALMETRICS – THE SOCIAL IMPACT OF SCIENCE

All these changes both in the new technological developments and the new ways of disseminating research outputs, have produced the appearance of new metrics that quantify the use and impact of these publications in these networking environments. The Almetrics Manifesto (Priem, Taraborelli, Groth, & Neylon, 2010) exposed the exhaustion of the classical assessment system, in which peer review and citations are slow, subjective and imprecise mechanisms of reward. Instead, altmetrics ensure a fast and collaborative way to 'filter' the most relevant scientific results thanks to the instant appreciation of these materials by a vast online community that comments, posts, votes, follows and downloads these results through the social platforms. Although the manifesto's authors cannot provide any evidence of this, they suggest that the computing of these measurements would provide an alternative to the traditional evaluation system. This document thus marked the starting gun for a broad range of studies to find the meaning of these metrics in the context of research evaluation. Thus, for example, tweets (De Winter, 2015; Eysenbach, 2011; Haustein et al., 2014a), Mendeley's readers (Bar-Ilan et al., 2012; Li & Thelwall, 2012), ResearchGate scores (Ortega, 2015) and paper downloads (Bollen, Van de Sompel, Smith, & Luce, 2005) were compared with citations. However, the results have not revealed any substantial relationships with the current bibliometric measurements and therefore it is hard to believe that they could be an alternative to the current bibliometric evaluation. Perhaps one of the problems is that the proposed almetrics include a wide range of heterogeneous metrics (tweets, views, downloads, posts, etc.) that describe very different actions and purposes (Brown, 2014), without distinguishing usage metrics from networking ones.

A further problem is that they are site-dependent, that is they are influenced by the environment in which they were created (Ortega, 2015). For instance, tweets are spread according to the number of followers a user has (Davis, 2012) and Academia.edu's views or Researchgate's downloads are determined by the number of users and publications in the network. Another problem is that these metrics are computed in environments external to the academic world. Tweets are dispersed in a popular network which appreciates the scientific results in a very different manner (Almetrics, 2014). One final problem is that these indicators are also time-dependent, as the more time a document is in the network, the more likely it is to be cited, shared, followed, etc. (Thelwall and Kousha, 2014). Surprisingly, in the midst of these unresolved problems and with clear evidence that these measures cannot be substitutes for the present system of evaluation, two firms, Almetric (2011) and ImpactStory (2011), the latter created by a number of the authors of the Almetrics Manifesto, emerged to provide statistics on these indicators for organizations and publishers. This uncovers a clear conflict of interest between commercial profit and scientific evidence, suggesting that there are more economic interests than scientific behind this movement (Colquhoun & Plested, 2014). In any case – and apart from the doubts that arise – the evidence of scientific studies is that these alternative metrics describe a very different effect, closer to the popularization of science or their impact on society than to research evaluation. In spite of this, this new generation of indicators is opening a window on the exploration of a new and different impact of science in environments far from the traditional publishing system. To some extent, these instruments bring to light the impact that the scientific literature exercises over scholars and professionals that are outside of the academic publishing system, a different and new world far from the classical bibliometric approach (Cronin, 2013).

1.5 SOCIAL NETWORK SITES FOR SCIENTISTS

Into the changing landscape of new communication developments, revolutionary transformations and controversial manifestos, a range of platforms for the benefit of scholars was born during the period 2006–8. Social sites for scholars have gained importance for the academic community because they bring together the issues described above. They support free and open access to the scientific literature, incorporate metrics that allow the tracking, impact and usage of these materials, and extend social networking beyond meetings, conferences and workshops to a virtual environment.

1.5.1 Definition

However, a clear definition of academic social sites is difficult because there is a varied range of platforms and services oriented to different types of actions. Moreover, there is no a clear agreement on how these sites are to be named. Thus *academic social sites* (Ortega, 2015), *academic social networking sites* (Goodwin, Jeng, & He, 2014; Gruzd, 2012), *academic social networks* (Almousa, 2011; Ovadia, 2014), *academic social networking services* (Jeng, He, & Jiang, 2015; Oh & Jeng, 2011) and *social media for academics* (Neal, 2012) are just some of the terms used to designate these sites. Nentwich and König (2014) put emphasis on the profile as the structural element and define social networking sites as the media that make possible the 'setting up a sophisticated personal "profile" with information about oneself, such as interests and activities, within a digital space that can usually only be reached after registration'. Calhoun (2014) used the generic term 'social web' to refer to 'the web sites, tools and services that facilitate interactions, collaboration, content creation and sharing, contribution and participation on the web'. Oh and Jeng (2011) state that 'academic social networking services' 'are online services (e.g. online platforms and/or software) that focus on supporting online research-oriented activities as well as building social networks for scholars', while Bullinger, Hallerstede, Renken, Soeldner, and Möslein (2010) describe it as 'a web-based service that allows individual researchers to (1) construct a public or semi-public profile within a bounded system, (2) articulate a list of other researchers with whom they share a connection and communicate, (3) share information with other researchers within the system and (4) collaborate with other researchers within the system.'

In our case, an approximate definition of the scholarly social site is formulated according to the essential capacities that they have to offer. Thus a social network site for scientists has to be an online space that generates statistics on its usage and the activity of its members contributing academic contents and interacting with other members. This definition considers four basic elements for building an academic social site: (1) *profiles* – through which a user can participate and interact in the network; (2) *contents* – the materials that are supplied or produced in the site; (3) *networking* – the connections that profiles make among them; and (4) the *metrics* –the measurements that quantify the actions performed in the platform. This last requisite is not indispensable but it constitutes a valuable object for the attraction of scholarly users. Hence content is at the centre of this definition because it is the instrument that articulates the relationship between the remaining elements.

1.5.2 Functions

In relation to the definitions above, several authors describe the principal functions that these platforms should develop. Codina (2009) describe three components: document management, academic profiles and groups. Bullinger et al. (2010) detect four main functions: identity and network management, communication, information management and collaboration. Oh and Jeng (2011) detail three basic functions: building a profile, management of personal publications and provision of a platform for online group research activities. Nentwich and König (2014) detail eight functions that a social site should accomplish: profiles, communication, networking, 'directing attention', groups, calendar, literature-related functions and further services. Many of them are easily dispensable nor are they exclusive to these vertical platforms. Espinoza-Vasquez and Caicedo-Bastidas (2015) found five actions that these sites must permit: collaboration, online persona management, research dissemination, documents management and impact measurement, and distinguished research dissemination and document management as services addressed to the contents contribution. In all these cases, these functions could be reduced to three basic types operations: a profile that identifies the user, instruments to put up and generate contents and an environment to share those outputs.

1.5.3 Motivations and Adoption

Many studies have approached the analysis of academic social sites from a qualitative point of view, exploring through surveys and questionnaires the perception of the academic community of these tools and the value they put on these sites for their research activities. A report from the Research Information Network (2010) defines two main benefits from the use of Web 2.0 services: communication with the research community and the support of colleagues in the use and adoption of new methods and techniques. Gruzd and Goertzen (2013) detected three benefits of using academic social sites: information gathering, collaboration and information dissemination. Other studies have discovered that in response researchers emphasize collaborative activities as the main benefit and utility (Jordan, 2014; Cann, Dimitriou, & Hooley, 2011). In this sense, Van Noorden (2014) revealed that most of the respondents used Academia.edu and ResearchGate for purposes of contact. Independent of these benefits, the ratio of adoption is quite low today (Procter et al., 2010) which could be cause by the absence of any immediate benefit, difficulty or reticence in the use of these platforms (Coppock and Davis, 2013). However, many authors have detected differences in adoption rates, mainly according to age (Park, 2010). In many cases, researchers adopt only one or two profiles at most in these platforms (Mas-Bleda, Thelwall, Kousha, & Aguillo, 2014; Haustein et al., 2014b; Ortega, 2015).

1.5.4 Typology

Social network sites for scientists are a heterogeneous set of applications that use different methods to promote interaction between their users. Bullinger et al. (2010) define four types of academic social network: research directory sites, research awareness sites, research management sites and research collaboration sites. Oh and Jeng (2011) just distinguish social networking sites from web-based social software. Nentwich and König (2014) distinguished different types of social network sites according to three criteria: intended usage forms, requirements for usage and available communication forms. In this study, academic social sites are grouped according the type of content and the way in which it is managed:

- *scholarly directories* – there are just lists of user profiles (i.e. BiomedExperts, UniPHY);
- *social bookmarking sites* – these are sites in which their users post and tag academic web resources (i.e. CiteULike, BibSonomy, Connotea);
- *reference management sites* – these are spaces where the principal activity is to share bibliographic references (i.e. Mendeley, Zotero, Qiqqa, Papers);
- *document sharing sites* – these platforms are addressed to share the academic outputs of their own users (i.e. ResearchGate, Academia.edu, Figshare).

1.5.5 Business Models

The building and start-up of an academic social site require an important economic effort that ensures the viability of the platform. Many of these sites started as student projects or experimental prototypes that requested funds from investors to initiate the first steps. Academia.edu, ResearchGate and Mendeley were financed by venture companies (Spark Capital and True Ventures), foundations (the Bill and Melinda Gates Foundation) and angel investors. The success of a site also has to be supported by a clear and defined business model that ensures its economic continuity (Peters, 2013). This does not mean that the model has to produce monetary benefits, but that the income must guarantee that the service will continue working with total normality. The importance of this fact is not founded on the site's own needs but on the fact that it contains items that many users have deposited and therefore the service should ensure access to these personal materials. Different approaches are used to gain income that makes possible the working of the network. Academia.edu opts to publish announcements of academic positions and, in the near future, will be offering an advanced stats service addressed to academic institutions to discover early impacted works (Shema, 2012). ResearchGate follows a similar approach with the publication of job offers supplied by Academic Jobs. Elsewhere, CiteULike is financed by ads from the AdWords service provided by Google as well as by subscriber members (gold) who pay for enhancing the storage space and access to specific services. Mendeley ensures its funds through an agreement with Elsevier as well as developing a paywall model for premium and institutional users who can access advanced functionalities. Meanwhile, BiomedExperts and UniPHY, developed by Collexis, were ending products that were sold as a block to academic institutions. Nature Network was a product entirely developed and supported by the Nature Publishing Group. Only BibSonomy and Zotero do not have a business model but are funded by academic organizations. These different business models are an example of the newness of these services and the difficulty of developing the optimal economic model for these products. In addition, several voices have set out ethical doubts on the monetary benefit of these platforms because they utilize user-generated contents for third parties to commercialize (Arvidsson and Colleoni, 2012; Fuchs, 2010). Other ethical problems arise when many of these services are constituted as private firms (i.e. ResearchGate and Academia.edu) that encourage open access, thus taking economic advantage of a public movement.

1.6 METHODS

The development of a quantitative study entails a precise and detailed description of the instruments, materials and sources used to extract and analyse the data.

1.6.1 Scope

This study is limited to a selected range of specialized social networking sites for scientists. Thus popular networking platforms such as Twitter, Facebook or Figshare, commonly used by researchers, were excluded because they do not specifically address the scholarly community. An analysis of these sites would show a distorted view of the academic activity and the results could not be narrowly representative of the scientific communication process. In addition, paywall systems such as EndNote were excluded because they limit access to non-customers. Google Scholar Citations was also excluded because, although it contains profiles, it lacks networking utilities. The two most representative sites from the previous typology were selected because of their popularity and their extensive use in the scholarly community. Two sites were selected to allow comparison. Thus BibSonomy and CiteULike were analysed as representative examples of social bookmarking sites, Mendeley and Zotero as reference managers and ResearchGate and Academia.edu as examples of document sharing sites. Nature Network and BiomedExperts are also described because they were pioneering platforms.

1.6.2 Indicators

Several indicators are proposed in this study (see below) to describe the performance of each social platform. One of the advantages of a quantitative approach is the ability to develop indicators that make possible measurement of the activity carried out by the network and thus make a fair comparison between platforms.

1.6.2.1 Activity

Activity refers to the proportion of items posted to the network by the number of users registered. Hence this indicator expresses to what extent users add content. This measurement is also calculated for groups and forums in contrast with the global activity on the platform.

1.6.2.2 Compound Annual Growth Rate

The compound annual growth rate (CAGR) is an indicator which measures the mean annual growth rate of a value across a time period. It is used to calculate the rate of increase of each social site according users, posts and publications. This measurement is most stable in exponential growths. The formula is:

$$CAGR(t_n,t_0) = \left(\frac{V(t_n)}{V(t_0)}\right)^{\frac{1}{t_n-t_0}} - 1$$

where V is the value in the initial moment (t_0) and in the final one (t_n). Commonly, it is interpreted in percentage terms.

1.6.2.3 Country Penetration

Country penetration is ratio of the percentage of users on a site and the percentage of researchers employed in R&D by country. This measure attempts to evaluate the success or failure of an academic site in a country.

The calculation allows a reduction of the size effect of large countries taking up scholarly social platforms. The information on the number of human resources appointed to scientific activities was obtained from the UNESCO Institute for Statistics (2015), being the last available data from 2011, although some countries only present data from previous years. This ratio of percentages was used because these statistics do not include all the scholarly community of a country since they exclude students and other professionals. It is thus presupposed that the proportion of those in R&D in a country could be similar to the total percentage of social network's profiles in that same country.

$$Penetration_{c,i} = \frac{\left(\dfrac{u_c}{U_i}\right)}{\left(\dfrac{n_c}{N}\right)}$$

In this way, penetration of a site (i) in country (c) is the proportion of users of that country (u_c) in the entire site (U_i) divided by the proportion of total researchers from that country (n_c) in the total amount of researchers in the world (N). A penetration beyond 1 shows that the proportion of researchers in that site is higher than the real world. Inversely, a penetration below 1 means that the site contains less researchers from a country in relation to the same proportion globally. The result is not a percentage and has to be interpreted as the number of times that one percentage is larger than another. For example, a penetration of 2.12 means that the percentage of users on a platform is 2.12 times higher than the same at world level.

1.6.2.4 Country Spreading

Country spreading (CS) is the accumulated percentage of users belonging to the first ten countries in each site. Thus a site with an elevated CS shows that the first ten countries contribute the majority of the users and, therefore, demonstrates that the site has not spread far. In contrast, a site with a low CS shows that there is a large number of users that belong to a range of countries which indicates that the site is globally spread. This metric allows us to make comparisons across platforms.

1.6.2.5 Recent Activity

This indicator tries to measure the percentage of content supplied during the period 2014–15. As more items are added to the platform in this period the more up to date and recent is the platform. This measurement allows us to observe sites that are becoming stagnant or spaces with strong energy.

1.6.3 Sources

In this study, a manual inspection of the respective social networks was undertaken to describe their functionalities and services. In particular, their blogs and help pages were retrospectively explored to find out when their functionalities were implemented or ceased. As much as possible, other sources such as bibliographies, scholarly databases and academic search engines were queried to gather the most exhaustive academic bibliography on these online services. A special mention is the use of the Archive.org WayBack Machine to find information on the evolution of these sites according users and documents. Archive.org is a non-profit organization that attempts to archive the most important pages on the Web. Thanks to the WayBack Machine, it is possible to explore successive snapshots of these pages across time, showing how these sites have evolved. On many sites, on the main page the number of registered users, number of documents, groups, etc., in that moment in time were frequently reported, so the WayBack Machine was considered a suitable tool to observe this evolution.

1.6.4 Data Extraction

A critical element in a quantitative analysis is the numerical data that describe the performance of the academic sites studied and the processes required to extract and harvest this information. Generally, several crawlers were designed to extract the desired data. Using a screen scraping technique, SQL scripts were written to navigate across the site architecture and extract the pieces of information needed for this study. 25 virtual machines from the Cybermetrics Lab were used to extract these data. In the case of BibSonomy, however, an API was used to extract information on users and posts. In other cases, such as Mendeley, these instruments offered limited possibilities and were discarded. In the case of services that have disappeared such as Nature Network and BiomedExperts several bibliographic sources were used to obtain a picture of their function and structure.

NOTE

1. Only English Wikipedia (2015).

REFERENCES

Almetrics, (2014). Almetric Top 100 – 2014. Available from: <http://www.altmetric.com/top100/2014/> Accessed 10.09.15.

Almousa, O. (2011). Users' classification and usage-pattern identification in academic social networks. 2011 IEEE Jordan conference on Applied Electrical Engineering and Computing Technologies (AEECT), 6th–8th December 2011, Amman, Jordan.

Arvidsson, A., & Colleoni, E. (2012). Value in informational capitalism and on the internet. *Information Society*, *28*(3), 135–150.

Bar-Ilan, J., Haustein, S., Peters, I., Priem, J., Shema, H., & Terliesner, J. (2012). Beyond citations: Scholars' visibility on the social Web, *arXiv preprint arXiv:1205.5611*.

Bollen, J., Van de Sompel, H., Smith, J. A., & Luce, R. (2005). Toward alternative metrics of journal impact: A comparison of download and citation data. *Information Processing and Management*, *41*(6), 1419–1440.

Boyd, D. M., & Ellison, N. B. (2007). Social network sites: Definition, history, and scholarship. *Journal of Computer-Mediated Communication*, *13*(1), 210–230.

Brown, M. (2014). Is almetrics an acceptable replacement for citation counts and the impact factor? *Serials Librarian*, *67*(1), 27–30.

Bullinger, A.C., Hallerstede, S., Renken, U., Soeldner, J.H., & Möslein, K. (2010). *Towards Research Collaboration – A Taxonomy of Social Research Network Sites*. Paper presented at the Americas Conference on Information Systems AMCIS 2010. Available from: <http://aisel.aisnet.org/amcis2010/92> Accessed 10.09.15.

Calhoun, K. (2014). *Exploring digital libraries: Foundations, practice, prospects*. London and Chicago: Facet Publishing and ALA Neal-Schuman.

Cann, A., Dimitriou, K., & Hooley, T. (2011). *Social Media: A Guide for Researchers*. London: Research Information Network. Available from: <http://www.rin.ac.uk/our-work/communicating-and-disseminating-research/social-media-guide-researchers> Accessed 10.09.15.

Castells, M. (2010). *The information age: Economy, society and culture volume 1: The rise of the network society* (2nd ed.). Oxford: Wiley Blackwell.

Codina, L.l. (2009). Science 2.0: Social networks and online applications for scholars, *Hipertext.net*, 7. Available from: <http://www.upf.edu/hipertextnet/en/numero-7/ciencia-2-0.html> Accessed 10.09.15.

Colquhoun, D., & Plested, A. (2014). Scientists don't count: Why you should ignore altmetrics and other bibliometric nightmares. *DC's Improbable Science* Available from: <http://www.dcscience.net/2014/01/16/why-you-should-ignore-altmetrics-and-other-bibliometric-nightmares/> Accessed 10.09.15.

Coppock, E. G., & Davis, L. (2013). Status of the adoption of social media in the scientific research community. *Information Services and Use*, *33*(3–4), 203–217.

Cormode, G., & Krishnamurthy, B. (2008). Key differences between Web 1.0 and Web 2.0. *First Monday*, *13*(6) Available from: <http://firstmonday.org/ojs/index.php/fm/article/view/2125/1972> Accessed 10.09.15.

Cronin, B. (2013). Metrics à la mode. *Journal of the American Society for Information Science and Technology*, *64*(6), 1091.

Davis, P. (2012). Tweets, and our obsession with alt metrics. *Scholarly Kitchen* Available from: <http://scholarlykitchen.sspnet.org/2012/01/04/tweets-and-our-obsession-with-alt-metrics/> Accessed 10.09.15.

De Winter, J. C. F. (2015). The relationship between tweets, citations, and article views for PLOS ONE articles. *Scientometrics*, *102*(2), 1773–1779.

Ellison, N. B., & Boyd, D. (2013). Sociality through social network sites. In W. H. Dutton (Ed.), *The Oxford Handbook of Internet Studies*. (pp. 151–172). Oxford: Oxford University Press.

Espinoza-Vasquez, F.K., & Caicedo-Bastidas, C.E. (2015). *Academic Social Networking Sites: A Comparative Analysis of Their Services and Tools*. Paper presented at iConference 2015 Newport Beach, CA. Available from: <https://www.ideals.illinois.edu/bitstream/handle/2142/73715/380_ready.pdf> Accessed 10.09.15.

European Commission. (2013). *Guidelines on Open Access to Scientific Publications and Research Data in Horizon 2020.* Available from: <http://ec.europa.eu/research/participants/data/

ref/h2020/grants_manual/hi/oa_pilot/h2020-hi-oa-pilot-guide_en.pdf> Accessed 10.09.15.

Eysenbach, G. (2011). Can tweets predict citations? Metrics of social impact based on Twitter and correlation with traditional metrics of scientific impact. *Journal of Medical Internet Research, 13*(4), e123.

Fuchs, C. (2010). Labor in informational capitalism and on the internet. *Information Society, 26,* 179–196.

Goodwin, S., Jeng, W., & He, D. (2014). Changing communication on researchgate through interface updates. *Proceedings of the American Society for Information Science and Technology, 51*(1), 1–4.

Gruzd, A. (2012). Non-academic and academic social networking sites for online scholarly communities. In D. Rasmussen Deal (Ed.), *Social media for academics: A practical guide.* Oxford: Chandos Publishing/Elsevier.

Gruzd, A., & Goertzen, M. (2013). Wired academia: Why social science scholars are using social media: *Proceedings of the 46th Hawaii International Conference on System Sciences.* Washington, DC: IEEE Computer Society.

Guédon, J. C. (2004). The "green" and "gold" roads to open access: The case for mixing and matching. *Serials Review, 30*(4), 315–328.

Harnad, S. (1994). *Publicly Retrievable FTP Archives for Esoteric Science and Scholarship: A Subversive Proposal.* The Network Services Conference (NCS), London, England, 28–30 November. Available from: <https://groups.google.com/forum/?hl=en#!topic/bit.listserv.vpiej-l/BoKENhK0_00> Accessed 10.09.15.

Harnad, S., Brody, T., Vallières, F., Carr, L., Hitchcock, S., Gingras, Y., et al. (2004). The green and the gold roads to open access. *Serials Review, 30*(4), 310–314.

Haustein, S., Larivière, V., Thelwall, M., Amyot, D., & Peters, I. (2014a). Tweets vs. Mendeley readers: How do these two social media metrics differ? *IT-Information Technology, 56*(5), 207–215.

Haustein, S., Peters, I., Bar-Ilan, J., Priem, J., Shema, H., & Terliesner, J. (2014b). Coverage and adoption of altmetrics sources in the bibliometric community. *Scientometrics, 101*(2), 1145–1163.

Jarvenpaa, S. L., & Todd, P. A. (1996). Consumer reactions to electronic shopping on the World Wide Web. *International Journal of Electronic Commerce, 1*(2), 59–88.

Jeng, W., He, D., & Jiang, J. (2015). User participation in an academic social networking service: A survey of open group users on Mendeley. *Journal of the Association for Information Science and Technology, 66*(5), 890–904.

Jordan, K. (2014). Academics and their online networks: exploring the role of academic social networking sites. *First Monday, 19*(11) Available from: <http://firstmonday.org/ojs/index.php/fm/article/view/4937> Accessed 10.09.15.

Knorr, E. (2003). 2004: The year of web services, *CIO Magazine.* Available from: <http://www.cio.com/article/2439869/web-services/2004--the-year-of-web-services.html> Accessed 10.09.15.

Li, X., & Thelwall, M. (2012). F1000, Mendeley and traditional bibliometric indicators. In É. Archambault, Y. Gingras, & V. Larivière (Eds.), *Proceedings of 17th international conference on science and technology indicators.* Montréal: Science-Metrix and OST.

Lieb, V. (2013). Setting the stage for Vertical Social Networks, *SlideShare.* Available from: <http://www.slideshare.net/lieblink/vertical-social-networks> Accessed 10.09.15.

Mas-Bleda, A., Thelwall, M., Kousha, K., & Aguillo, I. F. (2014). Do highly cited researchers successfully use the social web? *Scientometrics, 101*(1), 337–356.

Morris, M., & Ogan, C. (1996). The internet as mass medium. *Journal of Communication, 46*(1), 39–50.

Neal, D. R. (Ed.). (2012). *Social media for academics: A practical guide.* Oxford: Chandos Publishing/Elsevier.

Nentwich, M., & König, R. (2014). Academia goes Facebook? The potential of social network sites in the scholarly realm. In S. Bartling & S. Friesike (Eds.), *Opening science* (pp. 107–204). Springer International.

Odlyzko, A. (1997). The economics of electronic journals. *First Monday, 2*(8–4) Available from: <http://firstmonday.org/ojs/index.php/fm/article/view/542/463> Accessed 10.09.15.

Oh, J. S., & Jeng, W. (2011). Groups in academic social networking services – an exploration of their potential as a platform for multi-disciplinary collaboration: *2011 IEEE third international conference on privacy, security, risk and trust (PASSAT)*. Washington, DC: IEEE Computer Society. pp. 545–8

Ortega, J. L. (2015). Relationship between altmetric and bibliometric indicators across academic social sites: The case of CSIC's members. *Journal of Informetrics, 9*(1), 39–49.

O'Reilly, T. (2007). What is Web 2.0: Design patterns and business models for the next generation of software. *Communications and Strategies, 1*, 17.

Ostrow, A. (2011). Facebook now has 800 million users. *Mashable* Available from: <http://mashable.com/2011/09/22/facebook-800-million-users/> Accessed 10.09.15.

Ovadia, S. (2014). ResearchGate and Academia. edu: Academic social networks. *Behavioral and Social Sciences Librarian, 33*(3), 165–169.

Panitch, J. M., & Michalak, S. (2005). *The Serials Crisis*, Hill Scholarly Communications Convocation, UNC-Chapel. Available from: <http://www.unc.edu/scholcomdig/whitepapers/panitch-michalak.html> Accessed 10.09.15.

Park, J. H. (2010). Differences among university students and faculties in social networking site perception and use: Implications for academic library services. *Electronic Library, 28*(3), 417–431.

Peters, H. (2013). A quick glance at business models of academic social networking services: *Hybrid Publishing Lab: Researching News Form of Scholarly Communication in the Digital Age* Available from: <https://hybridpublishing.org/2013/01/a-quick-glance-at-business-models-of-academic-social-networking-services/> Accessed 10.09.15.

Priem, J., Taraborelli, D., Groth, P., and Neylon, C. (2010). *Altmetrics: A Manifesto*. Available from: <http://altmetrics.org/manifesto/> Accessed 10.09.15.

Procter, R., Williams, R., Stewart, J., Poschen, M., Snee, H., Voss, A., et al. (2010). Adoption and use of Web 2.0 in scholarly communications. *Philosophical Transactions of the Royal Society of London A: Mathematical, Physical and Engineering Sciences, 368*(1926), 4039–4056.

Research Councils UK. (2013). *RCUK policy on open access and supporting guidance*. Available from: <http://www.rcuk.ac.uk/RCUK-prod/assets/documents/documents/RCUKOpenAccessPolicy.pdf> Accessed 10.09.15.

Research Information Network. (2010). *If You Build It, Will They Come? How Researchers Perceive and Use Web 2.0*. Available from: <http://www.rin.ac.uk/system/files/attachments/web_2.0_screen.pdf> Accessed 10.09.15.

Shema, H. (2012). Interview with Richard Price, Academia.edu CEO: *Scientific American* Available from: <http://blogs.scientificamerican.com/information-culture/interview-with-richard-price-academia-edu-ceo/> Accessed 10.09.15.

Thelwall, M., & Kousha, K. (2014). Academia. edu: social network or academic network? *Journal of the Association for Information Science and Technology, 65*(4), 721–731.

UNESCO Institute for Statistics (2015). UIS.Stat. Available from: <http://data.uis.unesco.org/> Accessed 10.09.15.

Van Dijck, J. (2009). Users like you? Theorizing agency in user-generated content. *Media, Culture, and Society, 31*(1), 41.

Van Noorden, R. (2014). Online collaboration: Scientists and the social network. *Nature, 512*(7513), 126–129.

CHAPTER 2

The First Attempts

The first social platforms on the Web arose as exploratory services that were intended to create online academic communities using a range of basic tools that allowed connection between members. These sites were born as experimental platforms from different approaches. In some cases, there were services that concentrated their attention almost exclusively on communication tools about which users shared information and discussions (Nature Network). In other cases, the network was simply an expert database where users would be able to find other partners with similar research interests (BiomedExperts, UniPHY). However, in general, because these platforms were created from a pre-conceived and limited concept of online social networking they suffered from excessive intervention on the part of site administrators. Perhaps these corseted structures promoted the swift stagnation of these sites and in consequence their rapid closure. As will be seen, these pioneer services lacked many of the social networking instruments and offered little freedom of action; however, it should not be forgotten that they opened the path to the next generation of academic social sites, suggesting new forms of contact among scholars. The disappearance of these sites should remind us of the changing nature of the social web and that services that are successful today will soon become obsolete if they do not recycle the functionalities they offer to their users.

This chapter suffers the major inconvenience that every site analysed has now disappeared. The reason for this was that a major part of the information on these platforms was not taken first hand and was needed to gather external sources to describe these services. In many cases, it was not possible to access the site, while in other cases, a limited part of the site was only available. As a result of this, it is possible that the information on some sites could be somewhat incomplete and inexact.

2.1 NATURE NETWORK

Nature Network was the first web service that attempted to create a networked community of scientists around discussion groups and forums (http://network.nature.com/). It started life in February 2007 'as an

Social Network Sites for Scientists.
ISBN 978-0-08-100592-7

experiment in using social media for science' (Nature.com, 2013) from the Nature Publishing Group, responsible, among others, for the prestigious scientific journal *Nature*. In May 2010 the network was relaunched with the inclusion of new features such as a Q&A section and a Workbench. Its activity ceased in 2013, although the information on groups, forums and users is today accessible, having become a 'community archive' (Nature.com, 2013). The reason for its closure was not at all clear, although those responsible argued that it did not provide the level of service expected by the users.

2.1.1   A Wide Range of Contacting Tools

Nature Network presented several communication instruments at different levels. At the group level, the most relevant were Forums, Groups and Questions & Answers because they were meeting points where users could interact with each other and share information. Other services such as Blogs and the Workbench were addressed to the creativity of the users and their ability to spread information and contents. Otherwise, the Hub was the main instrument for connecting the network to real life though events and meetings.

2.1.1.1 Forums

Nature Network provided tools for establishing specialized forums where users could discuss issues and controversies on scientific advances. It contained 1,822 forums where 16,678 discussion topics were laid out. It is interesting to observe that three of the five most populated forums were promoted directly by the creators of the site themselves (i.e. *Nature India*, *Ask the Nature Editor* and *Careers Advice by NatureJobs*), which provides evidence of little incentive among this community to create its own active and dynamic forums. In general, the activity in these forums was quite low, with less than one (0.3) message per person and a participation rate of only 2.5 per cent of the Nature Network community (see Table 2.1).

Figure 2.1 shows the number of forums that posted their last message by year. In general, the distribution describes low activity, with a large proportion (66 per cent) of forums without messages two years before the closure. The linear trend of the cumulative distribution and the constant number of forums by year confirm that this application remained inactive.

2.1.1.2 Groups

This platform helped the creation of specialized groups in which the members were able to share papers, opinions and news on their research disciplines. With the exception of the sharing of documents, groups

Table 2.1 The five most active forums in Nature Network

Name	Members	Topics	Replies	Messages	Activity
Brain Physiology, Cognition and Consciousness	606	229	3,542	3,771	6.2
Nature India	1,386	1,336	2,296	3,632	2.6
Ask the Nature Editor	797	991	501	1,492	1.9
PhD Students	1,125	848	457	1,305	1.2
Careers Advice by NatureJobs	771	930	302	1,232	1.6
Total	**27,012**	**16,678**	**16,909**	**24,621**	0.9
Average	15.6	4.5	9.9	14.4	0.3

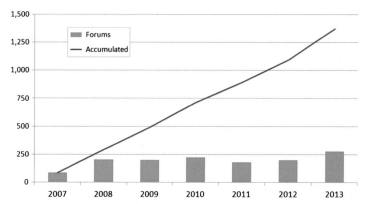

Figure 2.1 Number of forums by year in which the last message was posted in Nature Network.

technically worked as forums. In fact, participation in groups and forums was achieved through the same communication tools (topics and replies). However, this functionality was even less successful than in the forums – 188 different groups from psychology to scientific publishing were created (see Table 2.2), but the activity observed evidenced a low performance. Only an insignificant number of users (0.23 per cent) participated in these groups, with an average of 14.8 members per group. With the exception of *Brain Physiology, Cognition and Consciousness* (6.1), the rest of the groups presented less than one post per person.

2.1.1.3 Hubs

Nature Network had three hubs or seats in Boston, New York and London. Each location maintained bloggers, offered scholarly job vacancies and promoted social activities that were intended to give the virtual

Table 2.2 The five most active groups in Nature Network

Group	Members	Topics	Replies	Messages	Activity
Brain Physiology, Cognition and Consciousness	606	156	3,542	3,698	6.1
National Institutes of Health	275	13	12	25	0.1
NPG Libraries	157	43	53	96	0.6
GSAS Harvard Biotech Club	82	5	7	12	0.1
Science Commons	80	6	7	13	0.2
Total	2,792	501	3,761	4,262	1.5
Average	14.8	2.7	20.0	22.7	1.5

network to the physical world. The most active node was London with 71 topics and 156 replies, followed by New York with 55 topics and 235 replies and Boston with 44 topics and 35 replies. As in the case of groups and forums, the activities promoted by these hubs had scarce incidence in the community as only a small number of members replied.

2.1.1.4 Blogs
One of the most interesting features was that each user had the opportunity to build a personal blog into the platform. These enabled the diffusion of scholarly reflections and scientific news. The number of blogs that arose from Nature Network is unknown, but many were moved to SciLogs.com when the network closed. More than 25 blogs were moved to this new platform (Infotoday.com, 2012), but still a very low number for the total amount of users (approximately 1.3 million). In spite of this, it is commendable that this service was offered to the users because it encouraged the publishing spirit in their members to disclose scientific results. In fact, many of these blogs continued to work on the new platform without problem. Moreover, Nature's editors also developed personal blogs – 17 in total – that are still working on the Nature.com blog site.

2.1.1.5 Questions & Answers
The Questions & Answers (Q&A) section, added in 2010, allowed users to resolve any scientific question with the help of the online community (Nature.com, 2010). These answers were public and could be rated by the members according to their pertinence. The users that achieved better rates in their replies might be selected as Experts. Each profile would be

able to manage the list of questions launched to the community as well as the questions replied by the researcher him or herself. The questions could be sorted by time, rate and subject area. Unfortunately, all the information on this section was removed when the service closed in 2013, so it is not possible to track the number of questions launched or the rate of response.

2.1.1.6 Workbench

As with the Q&As, the Workbench was also released in 2010 (Nature Publishing Group, 2010). This original service enabled a customized view of the Nature Network by adding applications (widgets) that made it possible to search and share scientific information. These apps could be built on OpenSocial technology, allowing each user to develop their own gadgets and share them. For example, Nature Network developed some products such as tools for searching in Nature.com or inserting videos from the same site. It also promoted the use of APIs to design apps that needed data from other platforms such as Connotea.

2.1.2 The Natural Community

This last section is possibly the most important because it concerns the creation of a personal sketch in order to be able to participate in forums and groups. The main page talks of 25,000 colleagues but in December 2014 a crawling of the site estimated more than 1.3 million members. A sample of more than 800,000 profiles was obtained from that crawling, acquiring data on disciplines, organizations, countries, etc. This sample helps us to describe what kind of users shaped the Nature Network community. The first thing that attracts the attention was that most of the profiles do not include any information and only 32.1 per cent of the users filled the profiles with some data. For example, discipline is the section most filled out with 29.7 per cent, while group information is only presented in 1.6 per cent of profiles, affiliation in just 0.92 per cent, and sex and age in barely 0.5 per cent. This scant attention to filling out a personal profile is an example of the poor commitment of the users the site and it could be considered a qualitative measure of the success of these services.

In any case, although this information could be not representative of the 1.3 million Nature Network users, we could start from the hypothesis that users that include some information in their profiles would be motivated by a closer involvement with the site and a more active participation. In this way, data on disciplines, sex or age could describe the profiles of the most active users in Nature Network.

Table 2.3 Distribution of profiles by research area in Nature Network

Research areas	Profiles	%
Business/Investment	229,713	93.18
Other	6,318	2.56
Biology	4,066	1.65
Engineering	1,782	0.72
Chemistry	1,291	0.52
Medicine	1,263	0.51
Astronomy and Planetary Science	808	0.33
Earth and Environmental Science	769	0.31
Physics	504	0.20
Materials Science	3	0.00
Total	246,517	100

Table 2.3 shows the most frequent research disciplines in the Nature Network's profiles. Nature Publishing Group uses its own subject matter classification with which it arranges the content of its products. It is surprising that *Business/Investment* is the most frequent class with more than the 93 per cent of profiles. This could be due to some failure of assignation of that discipline and it is possible that it was added automatically by error. If that discipline is put to one side, *Other* (2.56 per cent) and *Biology* (1.65 per cent) are the disciplines that have the largest proportion of users in the system. Apart from *Business/Investment*, the distribution does not show any thematic bias and fits the common subject-matter distribution of large bibliographic databases (e.g. Web of Sciences, Scopus), although the elevated presence of *Other* could be a symptom of mis-classification or that the research activity of the users did not fit with that classification scheme.

By gender, Nature Network's population presents a high percentage of men (67.9 per cent) in contrast to the 32 per cent of women. This percentage is similar (30 per cent) to the percentage of women in science (UNESCO Institute for Statistics, 2015) which demonstrates that the participation in this network is the same for men and women. With regard to age, the average of age is 32.8 years old, which suggests that most of the users are young scholars at the start of their academic career.

Table 2.4 includes the five organizations with more profiles on the site. Universities prevail in the ranking, with Harvard University (2.64 per cent), Imperial College London (1.39 per cent) and Columbia University (1.38 per cent) outstanding. It should be pointed out that two of the universities with the most profiles come from United Kingdom, which evidences the strong presence of British users in the network. It is also

Table 2.4 Distribution of profiles by affiliation in Nature Network

Organization	Profiles	%
Harvard University	201	2.64
Imperial College London	106	1.39
Columbia University	105	1.38
University College London	100	1.31
Nature Publishing Group	87	1.14
Total	7,614	100

Table 2.5 Distribution of profiles by country in Nature Network

Country	Profiles	%	Penetration
United States	2,454	32.23	1.74
United Kingdom	1,156	15.18	4.08
India[*]	871	11.44	4.01
Germany	285	3.74	0.75
Canada	212	2.78	1.19
China	155	2.04	0.10
Australia[**]	139	1.83	1.33
Italy	125	1.64	1.04
France	113	1.48	0.40
Spain	91	1.20	0.62
Total	7,614	100	

[*]2010
[**]2008

surprising that the fifth organization by number of profiles is the Nature Publishing Group (1.14 per cent). This could be evidence of the strong support of the owner company for this platform, although it would also report an excessive intervention of this publishing group in energising the network.

Table 2.5 ranks the ten countries with the most users signed into Nature Network. The United States (32.2 per cent) and the United Kingdom (15.2 per cent) are the countries with the largest presence, followed by India (11.4 per cent) and Germany (3.7 per cent). On examination of the penetration index, the United Kingdom (4.1 per cent) and India (4 per cent) are the countries where this platform yielded the most success. This penetration is not surprising in the United Kingdom because the head office of the Nature Publishing Group is located in London (NPG, 2015). Perhaps more remarkable is the penetration in India, which could de due to influence of United Kingdom and the Anglo world as other commonwealth countries such as Australia (0.15 per cent) and Canada (0.13 per cent) show high penetrations as well. In any case, these results are not entirely representative of the total population in Nature Network and so may only be considered from an illustrative point of view. According to its distribution across countries, Country Spreading (CS) index shows that 74 per cent of users belong to the first ten countries, which suggests that the platform did not go beyond the British environment.

2.1.3 The Chatting Room

Nature Network was one of the first online social networks for scientists that permitted the building of personal and complete profiles as well as incorporating two fundamental communication tools (Forums and Groups) that made possible the interaction between users. These communication instruments can be considered group tools, that is applications that promote the interaction among users at the same time and in the same place. However, although these instruments were created with the purpose of building a large and cohesive community, the reality was that most of the users were not so much interested in those functions. Results from the crawler verified this fact. The participation degree in these services was quite low, with only 2.5 per cent of users involved in Forums and 0.2 per cent in Groups. If the activity inside these services is observed, data show poorer values with an average activity of 0.3 posted messages in Forums and 1.5 in Groups. The other instrument, the Blog service, only produced 25 logbooks. These figures are clear symptoms that the network did not come up to the expectations of the users and could provide the most decisive proof of the failure of this site. It is possible to reinforce this claim because, as a result of the low amount of information used to describe the profiles, only 32.1 per cent of them included any data.

One other cause that would explain the closing of the site was that the presence of the Nature Publishing Group in the network was evident at all times. Most of the active forums and groups were created and propelled by Nature staff which suggests that the company did indeed exercise a strong intervention in the network. Since most of the blogs were also published by members of Nature, a monitoring policy of the site was instituted aimed at fostering a community of loyal 'customers' interested in Nature products. However, it is also possible that this excessive intervention was caused by the low participation of its members, and in consequence the company was looking to somehow keep the site active.

Perhaps the last version introduced in 2010 incorporating the Workbench and Q&As could be understood as one final effort to stimulate the service. But the inactivity of the Forums and Groups sections and the scant information in the profiles decided in advance the eventual fate of the site.

In general terms, the Nature Network was the first initiative to pave the way to academic social sites with the sharing of information tools and personal profiles. However, it failed to create a comfortable environment that was attractive to the academic community. The model was closer to a chat room, in which direct communication between users in a public environment took precedence. Nature thus understood that a social network is just a public forum where research topics are discussed, recent publications are commented on and scientific news is spread. Nevertheless, any consistent virtual community should be based on the ability to produce and generate content which could then be shared, favouring networking and collaboration between its members.

2.2 BIOMEDEXPERTS

BiomedExperts was an initiative for creating an online community of experts in biomedicine and related sciences. It was produced by Collexis Holdings in 2006, an American leader in semantic search and knowledge discovery software. In 2010, the technology of the site was acquired by Elsevier. The platform was finally switched off in December 2014, being integrated into Mendeley, a bibliographic references-based social community linked to Elsevier. However, the technology is currently being used in Pure (before SciVal Expert), a commercial platform from Elsevier to design scientific information services for research organizations.

2.2.1 Scientist's Directory

Unlike other social services, BiomedExperts opted for automatically creating profiles as the starting point, thus counting on an initial population of profiles that gave consistency to the project. A key point in the success of an online social network is to have an important critical mass which allows its users to interact. As a specialized network in biomedicine, it started by creating 1.8 million 'knowledge profiles' from authors listed in about 18 million articles accessible through the PubMed database (BiomedExperts.com, 2011), the most important database on medicine. Only articles published during the previous ten years were selected to create profiles of active authors at that time. The authors of these profiles were then invited to participate in the network, edit their profiles more deeply and create new ties between their partners. However, BiomedExperts put up a number of restrictions when it came to creating a profile. Only users with a paper indexed in Pubmed within the previous ten years could create a full personal profile. Other users could simply browse the network of experts, but without any type of participation (BiomedExperts.com, 2010). This meant that the range of possible users was limited and most of them could only glance at the database.

The automatic creation of profiles of the authors of papers on the one hand produced duplicated profiles (i.e. distinctly different profiles corresponding to the same person) and on the other resulted in the merging of different authors with similar names. This is because researchers can author a research paper using different variations of their name. This problem is usual in academic bibliographic databases (e.g. Scopus, Microsoft Academic Search) and provokes inconsistency and noise (Ortega, 2014). In the case of social networks, it can cause mistrust and low performance. In BiomedExperts, each profile was disambiguated by identifying the 'fingerprints' of each author in keywords, places of work and age (Oswald, 2009) when it could not help but find duplicate and erroneous profiles.

However, in October 2014 there were only 473,000 profiles 'validated' by their respective authors (26.1 per cent), which informs us that interest from the research community was not very enthusiastic because only a quarter of the profiles were validated during the six years it had been running. To build the network, profiles were connected through bibliographical information, co-authors and research interests (Regazzi, 2013). In this way, any user could browse the network, jumping from one profile to another through any element the profiles had in common.

2.2.2 Interaction Tools

BiomedExperts, as a specialized directory of scientists, did not display any collaboration tools. Instead, it offered only a reduced range of communication tools. These could be divided into contacting devices at the profile level and instruments to assess articles. Thus each profile could only send internal messages to other members, bookmark researchers and add contacts to follow their updates and new publications. This reduced range of contacting tools limited the possibilities of user interaction, reinforcing the assumption that BiomedExperts was a scientific directory in which it was only possible to locate experts in specific fields and identify potential collaborators. In addition to this interaction function, there were other external tools that connected the network with other social sites. Thus it was possible to recommend a paper, profile or any other element through Twitter, Facebook, Connotea, etc.

At the publication level, it was possible to assess a paper (*Congratulate*), add it to a reading list or recommend it to other users. These mechanisms enabled the quality of a research paper to be evaluated, introducing impact elements into the publication list of a user. However, these instruments were limited to the publication list of a profile which could only gather articles from Pubmed.

2.2.3 Structure

As seen elsewhere, a user could only search partners and manage his or her own profile. The structure of the site was rather simple – just a display of a profile page from where other colleagues may be found and information on the user may be added. There were eight sections from the viewpoint of each user:

- *Home.* This part was devoted to the creation and management of the user's own profile.
- *Contacts.* This section listed the contacts added by each researcher and acted as an address book.
- *Messages.* This service made it possible to send internal mails to other profiles in the network.
- *Recent publications.* The most recent publications of a profile were included in this part. Note that BiomedExperts only included publications from Pubmed.
- *Reading list.* As a type of bookmark, this page included the articles authored by other profiles in the network, each having been selected as relevant or interesting for further study. The reading of these papers was possible if the user subscribed to the journal.
- *Find organization.* This element helped the search for organizations under which profiles were affiliated. It allows searching by name, keywords and places.
- *Find researcher.* As in the previous service, this section also included a search mechanism to retrieve profiles in BiomedExperts.
- *Conferences.* This last service showed conferences and events that might be of interest to the profile, with information on country, dates and deadlines.

2.2.4 Pre-elaborated Profiles

As said above, at the moment of closure it was claimed there were 473,000 profiles, far from the 1.8 million automatically pre-elaborated profiles. Using the WayBack Machine of Archive.org, it was possible to track the evolution of the number of validated profiles since 2010. Unfortunately, previous years did not offer information on this element.

Figure 2.2 presents the evolution in number of validated profiles for BiomedExperts since 2010, the first year in which that information is displayed in the home page, counting 258,000 users already registered. The distribution clearly describes a pattern of descent from 2011, the moment at which most users claimed their profiles. The annual growth rate is the lowest of the social sites analysed with an increase of 10.6 per cent each year. These results make clear the lack of success enjoyed by this platform with a constant reduction in new active users from 2011, three years following its creation.

Each profile (*Researcher Overview*) included a name and research topics (Figure 2.3). The only quantitative data were the number of publications and the members included in their personal network, detailing contacts at the first (*Co-authors*), second and third levels. Next, it presented the only networking functionalities on this site: send a message, add a contact and bookmark a profile. Below, there were six elements that gathered together the academic information on the profile:

• *Profile*. This section contained an exhaustive list of keywords that described the research topics of each author. These terms were

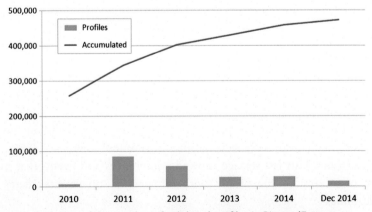

Figure 2.2 Evolution of the number of validated profiles in BiomedExperts.

extracted from the papers and came in turn from MeSH (Medical Subject Headings), the National Library of Medicine controlled vocabulary thesaurus used for indexing articles for PubMed. Behind each word, a bar described the frequency of profiles that included that term, providing a way to explore related researchers within that topic.

- *Publications.* This part listed the publications of each profile extracted from PubMed and sorted by publication date. BiomedExperts did not allow the management of those publications, so it was not possible to add or remove papers wrongly assigned by the system. Another problem was that it was not possible to add papers not indexed by PubMed. Each reference links to an article page which contained the abstract and MeSH terms.

- *Co-authors.* This tab contained the list of co-authors with one profile in BiomedExperts sorted by number of co-authored publications.

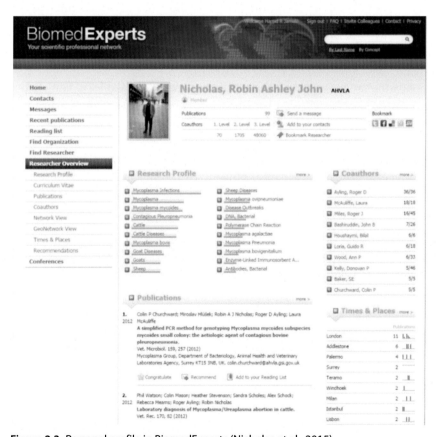

Figure 2.3 Personal profile in BiomedExperts (Nicholas et al., 2015).

- *NetworkView*. The last three sections corresponded to different visualizations of the co-author network. NetworkView graphed a circular ego-network with the first (co-authors) and second level of contacts. Several bars made it possible to refine the graph selecting the authors that most often collaborated (*Co-publications*) with the profile, most papers published (*Publications*) or most links had with other partners (*Connections*). On the right-hand side of the picture a full list of nodes was provided. The size of each name was proportional to the degree of collaboration. By clicking on each node, a short résumé of the profile was displayed.
- *GeoNetworkView*. This view showed the same co-author network but this time on a geographical map where each node was situated on a workplace. Red dots represented the workplace of the author, green the workplaces of the co-authors.
- *Times & Places*. This section described the cities in which their papers were published.

2.2.5 UniPHY: The Physics Sequel

Following in footsteps of BiomedExperts, in 2009 Collexis launched a similar product specializing in Physics for the American Physics Institute (AIP). UniPHY reproduced the same architecture as its big brother, creating a pre-elaborated population of 180,000 (300,000 in 2011) profiles from articles and papers published in 100 leading physics journals from Searchable Physics Information Notices (SPIN) in the previous 30 years as well as approximately 100,000 papers from scientific conferences (Seybold, 2009). However, its life was more ephemeral than its predecessor and it was closed in 2012.

2.2.6 A Static Network of Automatic Profiles

BiomedExperts and its younger brother UniPHY presented a particular strategy for creating an online community based on automatic profiles that were later claimed by their authors. In this way, Collexis could quickly generate specialized networks of researchers extracting authors from a large repository of scientific articles. These products were improved by means of a good semantic classification system that categorized each profile through relevant keywords. But, above all, the success of these social sites was due to their impressive visualization which became the key instrument for exploring profiles in the system.

However, while the collaborative relationships expressed in scholarly papers were the ties to build those networks, they were not the links that profiles established with other colleagues using contacting tools. BiomedExperts and UniPHY could not be considered online social networks because their architecture was not supported by the interaction of their users, but in the co-authorship network shaped outside the website. Although it is true that these platforms included contacting tools (adding a contact, bookmarking a researcher, etc.), these instruments were oriented to establishing further contacts through other media, not in the platform itself. In this form, Collexis' products were merely expert databases focused only on browsing and locating scholars, instead of platforms where the knowledge and expertise could be shared by the online community in the same place. This model produced passive profiles that were only used to show the research production of their users, more so if we take into account that two-thirds of the profiles were not edited by their authors. This model ended up as a static yearbook where the users were considered passive subjects that only showed their papers so they could be selected as partners.

A further factor that provided evidence that these products were not oriented to social networking was that the population of profiles was not only limited to disciplines, but to specific bibliographic sources such Pubmed in BiomedExperts and SPIN in UniPHY. This restrictive policy blocked the growth with new profiles and limited the publications that users could offer. To this may be added that these platforms were designed as isolated and specialized islands that did not represent the interdisciplinary nature of science. Perhaps this would explain why only one-third of their profiles were claimed in BiomedExperts.

In summary, the cause of the collapse of the Collexis model could be explained by a wrong understanding of the academic social networks, where users need a medium to share things, going beyond contact among them. This ignorance is also reflected in the restrictive conditions surrounding opening a profile, which meant a large proportion of researchers were not able to participate in the site.

2.3 WHY DID THESE SITES FAIL?

Nature Network and BiomedExperts were the two most outstanding initiatives of social networks for scholars. Both sites expected to build an online community from different approaches. In Nature Network, the engagement of the users with the system was established through groups and forums, the two principal social environments of the site. On the contrary, BiomedExperts and UniPHY were directories of scientists in which the interaction was channelled thought internal messages and follow-up contacts. This meant that some sites presented corseted structures that only permitted certain actions, making it hard for their users to develop a different activity than that pre-established by the system.

These limitations meant that these sites were characterized by an important interventionist attitude by the site creator, which directed user actions in specific directions. In the case of Nature Network, the most active groups, forums and blogs were those that were created by journalists and media professionals within the company. Perhaps this was an attempt to move the network and breathe new life into the project, though it could also generate a certain sense of control by part of Nature Publishing Group. Put another way, Collexis' products were closed environments in which even the profiles were automatically elaborated by the system. In addition, they had important restrictions on access, because only authors indexed in important databases such as Pubmed (BiomedExperts) and SPIN (UniPHY) could participate in the network. In this sense, while the service met the expectations of the owner in the creation of a directory of experts, it did not fulfil the desires of its users for sharing and generating content.

It is possible to think that this lack of flexibility in the architecture of these media was the cause of their inability to adjust to the users' requirements, gradually forcing the abandonment of these platforms. As has seen above, one of the critical elements in a social networking site is the possibility of producing content by the users themselves. In Nature Network, users could only share ideas and news by means of forums and groups, but they could not produce any content. One exception was the creation of a blog, but this tool required a great effort and only a very small number implemented this functionality successfully. In the case of Collexis' products, they did not even allow the addition of publications to the profile, much less initiate any discussion with other users.

In view of this inability to create content, these systems neither offered any metric that enabled the performance of a profile to be tracked nor made any action on the site possible. Thus users were not able to observe whether their actions or profiles were seen by other members. For example, Nature Network did not offer any information on visits to the profiles, nor even a rating of the responses in groups and forums. BiomedExperts only permitted congratulations on an article but without any account of the rewards. These restrictions brought about a lack of interest among users as the system did not pass on the impact or importance that these actions had for other users.

However, in spite of these important limitations which were the cause of the slow decline and later closure of these platforms, they were the first to introduce the idea of specialized social network sites for scholars. Today, it is inconceivable to think of an academic social site without a discussion space where scientific subjects are debated, or platforms without profiles that boost their publications and are connected through co-authors, interests or organizations. Both services contributed to laying the foundations for Science 2.0 and social networking in Science. As will later be seen, many of the current platforms owe a large debt to these pioneer sites.

REFERENCES

BiomedExperts.com. (2010). Terms of use agreement. Available from: <http://www.biomedexperts.com/Portal/ReadAGB.aspx> 15.01.15.

BiomedExperts.com. (2011). FAQ. Available from: <http://www.biomedexperts.com/Portal/FAQ.aspx> 15.01.15.

Infotoday.com. (2012). New home for Nature Network blogs. Available from: <http://newsbreaks.infotoday.com/Digest/New-Home-for-Nature-Network-Blogs-84031.asp> 10.09.15.

Nature.com. (2010). How to . . . use the new Q&A section, *Of Schemes and Memes Blog: A Community Blog from Nature.com*. Available from: <http://blogs.nature.com/ofschemesandmemes/2010/05/04/how-touse-the-new-qa-section> 10.09.15.

Nature.com. (2013). Nature Network becomes a community archive, *Of Schemes and Memes Blog: A Community Blog from Nature.com*. Available from: <http://blogs.nature.com/ofschemesandmemes/?p=9625> 10.09.15.

Nature Publishing Group. (2010). Nature Network extends OpenSocial "Workbench" for widgets, About npg. Available from: <http://www.nature.com/press_releases/workbench.html> 10.09.15.

Nature Publishing Group. (2015). Company information: about NPG. Available from: <http://www.nature.com/npg_/company_info/index.html> 10.09.15.

Nicholas, D., Herman, E., and Jamali, H.R., (2015). *Emerging reputation mechanisms for scholars*, JRC Science and Policy Report. Available from: <http://publications.jrc.ec.europa.eu/repository/bitstream/JRC94955/jrc94955.pdf> 10.09.15.

Ortega, J. L. (2014). *Academic search engines: A quantitative outlook*. Cambridge: Chandos Publishing/Elsevier.

Oswald, N. (2009). BiomedExperts: An alternative way to search the literature. *BitesizeBio* Available from: <http://bitesizebio.com/2331/biomedexperts/> 10.09.15.

Regazzi, J. J. (2013). *Infonomics and the business of free: Modern value creation for information services*. Hershey, PA: IGI Global.

Seybold, P. (2009). Creating a social network for physicists: AIP UniPHY. *Outside Innovation* Available from: <http://outsideinnovation.blogs.com/pseybold/2009/09/creating-a-social-network-for-physicists-aip-uniphy.html> 10.09.15.

UNESCO Institute for Statistics. (2015). Women in Science. Available from: <http://www.uis.unesco.org/_LAYOUTS/UNESCO/women-in-science/> 10.09.15.

CHAPTER 3

Social Bookmarking Sites

Under the influence of Web 2.0, many websites emerged with the purpose of building a community of users that feed the platform with their own creations. These in turn were organized according to the perception and valuation of the members themselves. In this form, this content could be set up for members without any mediation, from which emerged a self-organized and autonomous system. This structure was centred on the use of words for tagging the content supplied by the users themselves. These tags constitute the axis of the system because they are the main vehicle for browsing and searching these materials, in addition to having become the principal collaborative instrument. Following this model, dozens of sites, specializing in all sorts of content, arose across the web. Thus web platforms for sharing and tagging photographs (Flickr), videos (YouTube, Vimeo), presentations (Slideshare), links (Delicious, Reddit), etc., were born following this procedure.

This philosophy of building online social spaces where the content is organized by individual criteria was founded on folksonomy (Hayman, 2007). This concept of knowledge organization arose in around 2004 and advocated a system in which contents were directly and freely described by the users in natural language simply using keywords or tags. In some way, it intended to create a self-organized and universal knowledge system taking into account the individual perceptions of the persons. Its advantages are: its simplicity – no previous classification scheme is necessary, only tags that describe concepts; flexibility – there are no limits when it comes to assigning labels to an object; and findability – as more tags are used more the likelihood of finding an item. However, this system presents important limitations as well, for example: it is subjective – users may use contradictory words to describe the same object; there is no structure – because there is no previous scheme that relates these tags so there are no narrow and specific terms, no controlled language, polysemy, no plural/singular distinction, many words with a similar stem, etc. These problems make the retrieval of documents difficult and produce confusion and noise during the search (Marieke & Tonkin, 2006; Mathes, 2004).

Social Network Sites for Scientists.
ISBN 978-0-08-100592-7

Social bookmarking sites were born imbued with the spirit of the folksonomy and social tagging, proposing an alternative space where information was self-organized according to this model. At the same time, these platforms were aiming to create a collaborative environment which allowed discussion of, commenting on and valuing the posts of other members as well as producing collective products such as selected collections. In the academic environment, these sites offered the opportunity to create bibliographic services through the sharing and tagging of article references. These materials are the primary output of the research activity and it is essential they are informed in a discipline. So, it is not surprising that the social bookmarking sites for scholars rested upon these materials. Apart of this novel and relevant information model, social bookmarking sites favoured the establishment of an online academic community that took part in adding and tagging references, but also in valuing and discussing the impact of those items on the network. It is possible that these services appeared more as an alternative to other models of information management (i.e. search engines, directories) rather than as a place where a cohesive Science 2.0 community could be developed. In spite of this, they laid the foundations of the first social environment in which contents were the main goods for networking.

The first product of this nature was Connotea, a service launched by Nature Publishing Group in 2004, and was the first social medium addressed to scholars. It was closed in March 2013 due to growing problems with spam and associated service outages. Another ephemeral product was 2collab, a creation of Elsevier that was launched in 2007 and discontinued in 2011. CiteULike and BibSonomy were both born in 2006, are now the principal bookmarking services for scientists. This chapter will therefore focus on these two products as a way to explore the importance of social bookmarking for the scholarly community.

3.1 CITEULIKE

CiteULike is an online bookmarking service that helps to store, organize and share bibliographic references available on the Web. It was designed by Richard Cameron from the University of Manchester in 2004 for only private use. In 2006, Cameron was joined by Chris Hall, Kevin Emamy and James Caddy to set up Oversity Ltd, a company created to further develop and support CiteULike. In 2009, CiteULike signed an agreement with Mendeley to use the CiteULike library in the Mendeley desktop software (Mendeley blog, 2009). This is because CiteULike does not work as a reference management tool and it is not possible to insert references in any text. However, in February 2013, Mendeley stopped supporting the bridge.

CiteULike is a storage service of research references directed towards the academic community. It operates through a wide range of bibliographic formats that enable the automatic extraction of bibliographic records from any website and then their insertion in the library of each user thanks to a plug-in added to the web browser. This add-on software is a bridge that extracts the metadata of the source after including them in CiteULike. In this easy way users can feed their personal references database from any bibliographic source such as journals, repositories, citation databases, etc. It can extract/export citations from CiteULike itself, BibTex and RIS, which makes it compatible with reference management tools as well. Once the system extracts the bibliographic references, users can tag them in a natural language. In addition, these references can be edited to include more information such as external links to the original source or to upload a PDF file of the document. This turns CiteULike into a repository of researcher papers only accessible to the user him or herself.

3.1.1 A Decayed Database

One of the most successful aspects of this site is that it introduces a collaborative environment to enrich the value of the references posted. Created in the context of the folksonomies, Science 2.0 and social tagging, it develops a space where users can manage a wide list of references in touch with others, creating a great virtual library which organized through the individual actions of its users. In this way, CiteULike attempts to generate a large bibliographic service where the information is classified and organized thanks to the particular decisions of its members.

Figure 3.1 plots the number of articles posted to CiteULike and its accumulative curve. WayBack Machine from Archive.org was used to extract these data, but unfortunately CiteULike did not start publishing these data until 2008. In total by March 2015 CiteULike had reached 8 million papers uploaded to the system. The columns describe a general drop in the number of documents added annually, describing a slowing down in posting activity. The general annual growth was 19.5 per cent though during the last five year this has dropped to 7 per cent. These results provide evidence that the posting activity was already slowing down in CiteULike from 2008.

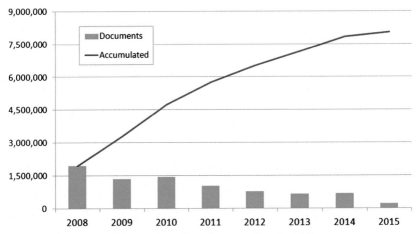

Figure 3.1 Evolution of the number of articles posted to CiteULike.

3.1.2 Building a Social Library

CiteULike operates using various social instruments to ensure the interaction of its members and the contribution of content. In this sense, two types of social tools can be differentiated, those that are addressed to the bookmarking of documents (groups, tags, watchlists) and those that are exclusively oriented to contact between users (blogs, connections). The first are instruments that support the creation and organization of a library from the previous actions of other users. With the exception of Groups, these elements are not collaborative but generate public results that can be taken advantage of by other users when they come to create their own libraries.

3.1.2.1 Tags

CiteULike employs a document classification system based on the use of tags or keywords created freely by their users. Each tag can be used again by each user, generating a participative process in the organization of papers named folksonomy. This system has the advantage that it does not need a previous scheme and the tags directly reflect the perception of the users of the document content. On the contrary, the use of labels or tags generates many terms that have similar meaning and ought to be processed (stemming) to analyse their vocabulary. In addition, these keywords do not belong to any scheme so it is not possible to build hierarchical relationships between broad and narrow terms.

Table 3.1 The ten most frequent tags in CiteULike

Tag	Frequency	%
Elegans	55,536	0.78
c_elegans	55,528	0.78
Nematode	55,528	0.78
caenorhabditis_elegans	55,523	0.78
Celegans	55,520	0.78
Wormbase	55,518	0.78
meeting_abstract	27,389	0.38
Article	15,750	0.22
Diatomics	8,962	0.13
Unassigned	8,962	0.13
Total	7,149,443	100

Tags illustrate to some extent the thematics of the document posted and the most active users from a disciplinary point of view can be observed. Table 3.1 shows the ten most frequent labels extracted from CiteULike in March 2015. The six most frequent terms are related to the nematode c. elegands, an organism studied in developmental biology – as such, it seems that biologists are the most active members posting documents. However, these tags have the same frequency because they are used by a very active group, *C. elegans/WormBase*, most of whose papers have been uploaded to CiteULike. This also shows that the use of tags is very varied without a clear thematic pattern. For example, from a sample of 444,233 tags, 71 per cent were used less than ten times, which suggests a low rate of tags per document (Good, Tennis, & Wilkinson, 2009). The next most used tags, *meeting_abstract* (0.38 per cent) and *articles* (0.22 per cent), are transversal tags without a thematic sense but related to the typology of the documents.

3.1.2.2 Groups
Another section linked to the collaborative posting of documents is Groups, a social tool addressed to put users in contact through their own libraries. Each group acts as a shared and open library in which each member can post references and tag them. In addition, members may interact between themselves by sending internal messages, holding discussions through a forum and publishing the results in a blog. There were 5,085 groups identified, from which 28,990 (13.9 per cent) users were inscribed in at least one group (Santos-Neto, Condon, Andrade, Iamnitchi, & Ripeanu, 2014).

This percentage is rather low and suggests that this social tool is not attractive to the majority of the users. In fact, only 55 per cent of the groups have more than one user. On average, each group consists of 5.7 members, the same number as in 2008 (Lee & Brusilovsky, 2010), which suggests that many of these are old groups and that no new users have joined them recently.

Figure 3.2 shows the number of groups by the year in which they posted their last paper as an indicator of the degree to which group activity is updated. The annual columns describe a descending trend since 2008, which confirms the general drop in performance of the service viewed earlier (see Figure 3.1). Since 2010, half of the groups show no action, with the years 2008 and 2009 having the most activity (12 per cent). In addition, from 2014, only 11.3 per cent of the groups show any activity. These figures suggest that the Groups utility is falling into disuse and many are becoming inactive. Another significant fact from this decline in CiteULike's groups is that since the creation of the platform, the number of groups has increase annually by 42 per cent, but in the last five years this creation rate has drastically fallen to 7 per cent.

Only 538,921 (8 per cent) papers are posted to these groups, a rather low proportion that again confirms the poor success of this social functionality and suggests that CiteULike is mainly used for private purposes. It is also interesting that 1,093 (21.5 per cent) groups do not include any documents. However, 106.3 papers on average were posted to these groups, an average much higher than that found in Profiles (25.7). This

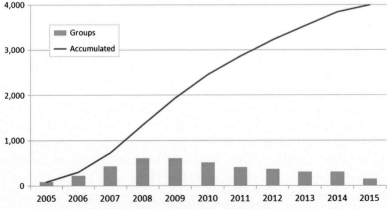

Figure 3.2 Number of groups by year in which the last post was made in CiteULike.

means that, although these groups are not numerous, they are very active in uploading references.

This activity contrasts with the lack of use of communication tools included in Groups. For example, each group has a forum in which group's members can open threads when posting comments and generate discussions. However, the number of threads in these communities is only 2,427, 0.4 threads on average, reflecting that these groups are not used to discuss or comment on any information. Moreover, the group *CiteULike-discussion*, used as place for reporting bugs and solving usage problems, collects 2,220 threads, 91.5 per cent of all the threads in the system. This means that the use of forums is almost non-existent. Another communication tool in Groups is blogs. The purpose of this service is for news to be posted or any other text that helps the group working. These comments may be open or closed according to the type of group. As with forums, blogs are even less used. Only 114 (2.2 per cent) blogs with any posts were located and 63 per cent of them had not had any new content since 2010, which indicates that the blogs are anecdotal tools with a very low performance.

Table 3.2 presents the groups that contain most documents. As it was seen before, *C. elegans/WormBase* (5.15 per cent) is the most active group

Table 3.2 The ten most important groups by number of documents uploaded

Name	Documents	Members	Activity	% documents	Type
C. elegans/WormBase	27,741	29	956	5.15	Open
Computational Cognitive Neuroscience Lab	16,363	3	5454	3.04	Applying
Journal picks	9,963	81	123	1.85	Applying
biodiversity_ conservation	6,599	100	65	1.22	Open
HEIRS – Environmental Illness Research	6,427	18	357	1.19	Open
PARDEM	6,276	30	209	1.16	Applying
T-MAPPP	6,255	7	893	1.16	Applying
Climate Change and Forests	4,926	2	2463	0.91	Invitation
Bioinformatics	4,529	245	18	0.84	Open
FAB-lab	4,300	8	537	0.80	Applying
Total	538,921	28,990	18.6		
Average	106.3	5.72	32.6	0.48	

uploading documents, followed by *Computational Cognitive Neuroscience Lab* (3.04 per cent) and *Journal picks* (1.85 per cent). It is interesting to note that the distribution of users in these groups is very different, with very populated groups such as *Bioinformatics* (245) and *biodiversity_conservation* (100), and small sets with just a few of members such as *Climate Change and Forests* (2) and *Computational Cognitive Neuroscience Lab* (3). This suggests that the reasons for creating a group are very varied and arise from a wide range of needs. Thus there are groups built from a purely thematic view such as *C. elegans/WormBase* and *Computational Cognitive Neuroscience Lab* which attempt to create specialist libraries on specific issues. Other groups, such as *PARDEM* and *T-MAPPP*, emerge as supporting tools for research projects, delivering a basic library that helps the accomplishment of their tasks. In other cases these groups have an institutional origin, such as *Journal picks* (Wellcome Trust Sanger Institute) and *FAB-lab* (Simon Fraser University), whose function is to coordinate an update bibliographic collection for their research staff. Although the *PARDEM* and *T-MAPPP* groups are devoted to Physics and Computational methods, the rest of groups in the list are related to Biomedicine and Environmental Sciences, which seems to suggest that biologists and biomedical researchers are more likely to create groups in this networking service.

3.1.3 A Community in Decline

CiteULike includes a profile for each user in order to identify their members in the network and these can take part in any bibliographic group. These profiles comprise valuable information about location, position, affiliation, date joined and research fields that assists in the description of the distinctive features of this community. During March 2015, a crawler was developed to extract the most exhaustive list of profiles. An initial strategy was to select profiles by Research Fields, because this part is mandatory and all users have to be listed there. However, the system does not display more than 2,500 users by category, so not all the profiles in large disciplines can be retrieved. Another limitation is that this classification was not incorporated until 2010, meaning that users that joined the service before that date could be not listed. Thus a complementary crawler was designed to randomly select profiles from Everyone's Library, a place where the most recent posts are listed. Finally, a total number of 208,243 profiles were retrieved. The representativeness of the sample was tested comparing with previous studies. For example, Emamy and Cameron (2007), creators of the site, detailed that there were 33,000 users in 2007, while the present sample contains only 17,582 (53 per cent) for that year. This disparity could be explained because pre-2010 profiles cannot be retrieved if they do not post an article, so this number actually corresponded to users that posted any papers. Emamy and Cameron (2007) also detailed that only 45 per cent of the users had posted a paper, a figure close to the 53 per cent found by the recent crawler. In consequence, this sample contains a proportion rather close to that of Emamy and Cameron (2007). Another study (Santos-Neto et al., 2014) detected 40,327 profiles in 2009, while the present sample contains 38,336 (95 per cent) at that date. However, Jiang, He, and Ni (2011) found 87,174 profiles in December 2010, 33 per cent less than our sample. Taking these reference figures into account, we would suggest that this sample is not greatly different to the others and may be representative of the total population of CiteULike.

Figure 3.3 shows the total number of profiles retrieved and grouped by joining date. It describes a regular increase in profiles from 2004 up to 2009, with a little gap between 2007 and 2009 that could be motivated by the extraction problems mentioned above. Then, a sudden jump occurs between 2009 and 2010 where the population is doubled, being the year with most profiles. However, since 2010 the ascription of new users gradually falls each year with only 17,730 new entries in 2014. The annual growth rate proves this fact, observing a total growth of 84.1 per cent in the entire period, but only 9.8 per cent during the last five years. This trend coincides with the drop of activity previously observed in Groups, confirming that this drop of activity is not exclusive to profiles but occurs in the whole site in general.

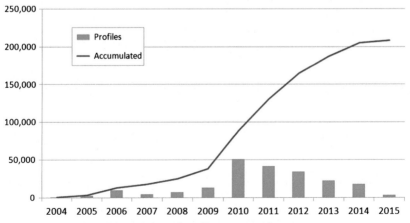

Figure 3.3 Evolution of the number of profiles in CiteULike.

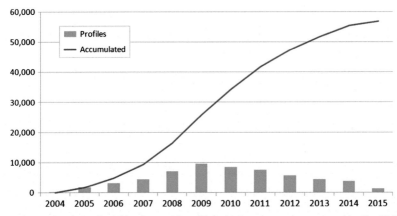

Figure 3.4 Number of profiles by year in which the last paper was posted in CiteULike.

Another way to observe the evolution of the activity on the site is to measure when their users stopped posting documents. This could be an indicator of when they gave up being interested in the site. Figure 3.4 shows the number of users by the year in which they posted their last paper. Since 2004, the posting activity appreciably increases till 2009, which saw the highest number of posted papers (Bogers & Van den Bosch, 2008). From that point, activity decreases more and more to the present. In general, this slow decline since 2009 could indicate a gradual loss of interest in this site by part of the scientific community due perhaps to the emergence of new, more advanced competitors or the obsolescence of many of their developments.

An important method to measure the activity in CiteULike is to observe the effort of users make in posting references into their personal libraries, to illustrate user interest in using platform. Figure 3.5 graphs on a logarithmic scale the distribution of papers by user. It follows a power law trend with a low exponent ($\gamma = 1.66$), which means that the differences between users are not very high. In fact, only 25 per cent of the users have any documents in their libraries and of these 45 per cent host less than ten papers. These results describe a low use of the libraries and suggests that only a small number of users are using this function to a great degree.

According to the academic position of the profiles, 139,333 (66.9 per cent) users included information on this aspect (see Table 3.3). Many of these were *Not Specified* or *Others* (59.2 per cent), so only 41.9 per cent included specific information on their scholarly posts. This distribution

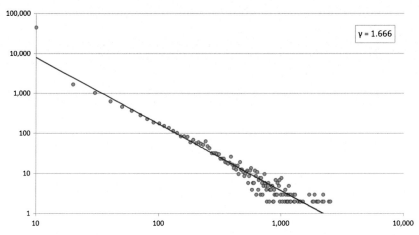

Figure 3.5 Binned distribution of posted references by user in CiteULike (log-log plot; bin = 10).

Table 3.3 Distribution of profiles by academic position

Position	Profiles	% Profiles
Graduate Student	24,428	17.53
Undergraduate Student	13,039	9.36
Researcher	4,415	3.17
Professor	3,660	2.63
Lecturer	2,962	2.13
Assistant Professor	2,629	1.89
Associate Professor	2,169	1.56
Reader	1,771	1.27
Postdoctoral Researcher	1,736	1.25
Research Fellow	1,555	1.12
Total	139,333	

also indicates, in an approximate way, the academic age of the users. The most frequent categories are *Graduate Student* (17.5 per cent) and *Undergraduate Student* (9.36 per cent), which correspond to young scholars at the start of their research careers. On the other hand, *Researcher* (3.2 per cent) and *Professor* (2.6 per cent) are academic staff that have an established scholarly activity. These figures illustrate that the service is preferred by young researchers who are preparing their doctoral dissertations or are starting their publishing career. This could be because in this point,

Table 3.4 The ten countries with most users in CiteULike in 2015

Country	Profiles	% profiles	Penetration
United States	2,619	27.23	1.47
United Kingdom	1,033	10.74	2.89
India*	459	4.77	1.67
Germany	445	4.63	0.92
France	384	3.99	1.08
Brazil*	362	3.76	1.83
Spain	326	3.39	1.76
Canada	321	3.34	1.43
Italy	313	3.25	2.07
Australia**	291	3.03	2.21
Total	9,619	100	

*2010.
**2008.

researchers need to be informed of other work in their respective research fields and check the most recent literature. Thus it is natural that students would be the users most interested in this type of platform.

Finally, Table 3.4 presents the ten countries with the highest number of profiles in CiteULike. Only 9,619 (5 per cent) users included information on their location or affiliation, so these results have to be considered for informative purposes only. This low proportion could be due to the fact that many of them are students, and do not have a definite institutional affiliation. Otherwise, it is possible that this information is not relevant when it comes to sharing bibliographic references and was not filled in most cases. In any event, Table 3.5 shows that users mostly come from the United States (27.2 per cent) and the United Kingdom (10.7 per cent), the country where the service was born. It is not surprising that the highest penetration index is for the same country (2.9), followed by Australia (2.2) and Italy (2.1). In general, the distribution of users by country suggests that this platform is better entrenched in Commonwealth countries. The Country Spreading index shows that 68 per cent of users came from the first ten countries, which suggests a wide diffusion of the service to the entire world.

3.1.4 Research Fields

In 2010, a classification system was incorporated to thematically group the members, with the aim that users might find and contact other members with similar interests. CiteULike uses the Joint Academy

Coding System (JACS) (HESA, 2015) for classifying the research interests of their users. This hierarchical scheme is structured on three levels,
but CiteULike groups these levels into two subsections, selecting certain
classes and omitting others. It is mandatory for each user to select at least
one research field as primary and then select other fields as secondary.
A crawler launched in March 2015 extracted a list of users by research
field. However, CiteULike only shows the first 2,500 users by field, so
in some cases the total value was estimated. As seen above, this classification was added in 2010, so a high proportion of users may not have been
classified. The fields with most users are *Biological Sciences* (14.6 per cent)
and *Medicine and Dentistry* (11.3 per cent), whereas the smallest fields are
*Eastern, Asiatic, African, American and Australasian Languages, Literature and
Related Subjects* (0.5 per cent) and *European Languages, Literature and Related
Subjects* (0.4 per cent) (see Table 3.5). These percentages show that biologists and biomedicine researchers have a strong presence in this space,
which could explain why these users are the members that most groups
create and are the most active tagging papers.

Table 3.5 Distribution of profiles by research fields

Research fields	Total	%
Biological Sciences	32,974	14.61
Medicine and Dentistry	25,574	11.33
Education	25,255	11.19
Mathematical and Computer Sciences	21,837	9.68
Business and Administrative Studies	20,099	8.91
Engineering	20,050	8.88
Social Studies	19,439	8.61
Physical Sciences	13,744	6.09
Subjects Allied to Medicine	8,184	3.63
Technologies	7,088	3.14
Creative Arts and Design	5,473	2.43
Mass Communications and Documentation	5,029	2.23
Historical and Philosophical Studies	4,627	2.05
Architecture, Building and Planning	4,618	2.05
Law	3,372	1.49
Linguistics, Classics and Related Subjects	3,210	1.42
Veterinary Sciences, Agriculture and Related Subjects	3,208	1.42
Eastern, Asiatic, African, American and Australasian Languages, Literature and Related Subjects	1,081	0.48
European Languages, Literature and Related Subjects	820	0.36
Total	225,682	100

3.1.5 The Decay of an Extended Service

CiteULike has become the most representative example of social book-marking sites for the scholarly community because it has brought together the most extended community of members (more than 200,000 users) and covers all the main research areas. In this sense, it could be said that CiteULike contains a representative sample of the scientific community with an important presence of biologists (14.6 per cent) and physicians (11.3 per cent). On the other hand, it also describes a balanced geographical distribution, although some of the best represented countries are from the Commonwealth. However, this platform also contains an important but disproportionate presence of graduate and postgraduate students (26.8 per cent), many of them perhaps attracted by the possibilities for uncovering new and updated bibliographic references.

Another relevant feature of CiteULike is that the social interaction is not limited only to sharing content through tags and groups, but it also aims to create a real networking environment where it is possible to discuss opinions on uploaded references or publish results obtained from these references. However, the analysis of these social tools demonstrates that most of the users are not interested in collaboration tasks. For example, only 13.9 per cent of users are linked to some group, who post just 8 per cent of the total number of documents in the system. On the other hand, the activity in these groups (32 posts/user) is slightly greater than in the site overall (26 posts/user), which suggest that members linked to groups are more active than the profiles not affiliated to groups. On the other hand, blogs and forums are instruments designed to get along with their members and share information and knowledge. Nevertheless, these instruments are underused and rejected by most group members. Forums are inexistent and only 2 per cent of groups have a blog. These figures illustrate that most of the users prefer to employ CiteULike for private purposes (i.e. managing their own library) rather than to participate in collaborative tasks with other members. In this sense, this networking space is not achieving the creation of a dynamic and participative community, but rather a platform for isolated users focused on their own interests.

However, CiteULike has been experiencing a generalized decline since 2009. From that moment the number of new users began to plummet, as did the rate of last posts in both groups and individuals. In terms of any parameter, CiteULike is losing performance and is in danger of stopping or disappearing. The reasons for this absence of vigour are varied. The most important could be its limitations as a reference management tool. As a bookmarking tool CiteULike is a good instrument but it fails when it comes to the management of this library such as its integration into written documents and the generation of bibliographies (Gilmour & Cobus-Kuo, 2011). This situation was highlighted by the Mendeley agreement in 2009, which may have provoked a migration to new software with more bibliographic solutions. In general, the appearance of the networking functionalities in reference management and document sharing sites would relegate CiteULike to a marginal and secondary position, as well as evidencing the obsolescence of its model and the need to adapt to the new networking trends in scholarly social sites.

3.2 BIBSONOMY

Another important bookmarking tool is BibSonomy, a service developed by a mixed group of German scholars from the Institute of Knowledge and Data Engineering at the University of Kassel, the DMIR group at the University of Würzburg and the L3S Learning Lab Lower Saxony in Hannover (Wikipedia, 2015). This service started as a student project in spring 2005 and quickly grew out of the prototype status into definitive release in 2006. In 2007, BibSonomy signed an agreement with the Digital Bibliography and Library Project (DBLP) to automatically import references from this database (BibSonomy blog, 2007).

As with other services dedicated to the online bookmarking of information resources, BibSonomy is a platform where users can upload any type of document to be shared with the scholarly community brought together in this service. These materials can be freely tagged by any member using labels taken from natural language without any type of limitation. In fact, in order to improve the findability, the system developed a recommendation mechanism to suggest tags. In this way, the more an item is tagged the easier it is to find it.

An interesting feature of BibSonomy is that it distinguishes between posting bibliographic references (publications) and other material accessible via the Web (bookmarks). In this sense, BibSonomy is somewhere between a classical bookmarking tool such as Delicious or Digg and an online citation service such as CiteULike and Connotea. There are different ways to include a document in the platform. The first is to directly post the item by filling out a form, which can be automatically completed inserting only the ISBN, ISSN or DOI of the document. The other way is through a plug-in in the web browser that directly captures the metadata of the object. These references can be processed through JabRef, an open reference management system that enables the building of bibliographies and insertion of citations in research papers. BibSonomy stores the bibliographic references in BibTeX format so users can export records to any other reference management tool such as EndNote and ReferenceManager and in any output such as HTML, RIS, CSL or MS Office XML. In addition, it is possible to add a full-text paper linked to a publication, although this file is only visible for users themselves and their friends or groups. This allows the creation of personal repositories of articles.

3.2.1 Coverage, a user Called DBLP

Figure 3.6 shows the distribution of items posted by year. BibSonomy has an API at the user's disposal to find data on the service and to automatically post high volumes of items to the network. Thanks to this API 3.45 million references were identified, from which 3.02 (87.7 per cent) were publications and 0.42 (12.3 per cent) web resources. This confirms that there is a great difference regarding to the type of material posted to BibSonomy, demonstrating that most of the items uploaded are bibliographic references (Borrego & Fry, 2012). However, the platform signed an agreement with the DBLP in 2007 according to which the latter database supplies bibliographic references to be directly posted in BibSonomy. These publications are included by the user *@dblp* and tagged with *dblp*, so these materials can be retrieved with a query selecting those parameters.

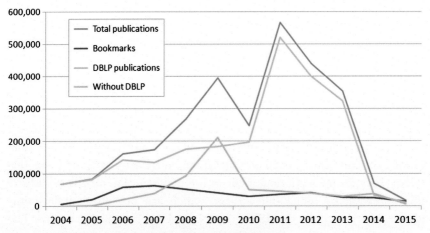

Figure 3.6 Evolution of the number of items to BibSonomy.

Figure 3.6 also shows that the majority of the bibliographic references, 2.33 million (76.9 per cent), posted to BibSonomy come from the DBLP. Subtracting the posts from that bibliographic database, the number of citations uploaded by the users would be then 0.69 (23.1 per cent) millions. Although the proportion of publications is still higher than with bookmarks, the difference is now not so high. Figure 3.6 describes a general increase in publications and bookmarks from 2005 to 2011. From that point, the number of new posts drops abruptly with an annual growth of 27 per cent that has fallen to 12.9 per cent in the last five years. When it comes to posting resources this could be symptomatic of loss of performance on the site. The graph also shows an activity peak in 2009. This could be due to the ECML PKDD Discovery Challenge, an event held in 2009 where several members posted and tagged items to test the reliability of the system (BibSonomy Blog, 2009). This punctual event demonstrates that the activity in adding references to the system is low because this performance caused a marked footprint in the evolution of the posting activity in the service.

3.2.2 The German Club

Any user has to be registered for posting and tagging papers and web resources in BibSonomy. This allows each member to be identified and makes interaction with other users and collaboration in groups possible. Through the API, it is possible to determine the total number of users that participate in the service. Thus 918,705 users were identified in this way, but only 8,947 (0.97 per cent) of them posted any document to the network. The high percentage of inactive users could be to unsubscribed users deciding to leave the site or simply users that do not take part in the platform. In any case, it could indicate a sign of dissatisfaction with the system.

Among the active members, there are more users posting publications 6,252 (68.9 per cent) than bookmarks 4,803 (53.6 per cent). In addition, 545,595 bibliographic records were uploaded to the system, a proportion of 87.3 papers by user, while only 335,172 bookmarks, 69.8 per member, were posted. These figures are lower than the previously observed total number of publications and bookmarks in the system. It could be that the site only shows the number of posts up to a certain point. Hence, for example, there is no count of the number of publications posted by the user *@dblp*, the largest contributor to the platform.

With regard to the origin of these users, BibSonomy allows the building of personal CVs where members may put basic identification data and list their own publications. However, this is anecdotal because only 347 users include any data on their curricula, a derisory percentage of 3.8 per cent. Analysis of these curricula provides only an approximate view of the total users that participate in the site. According to the location and affiliation of these curricula, it is worth highlighting that 41 per cent come from Germany, 7.2 per cent from the United States and 4.6 per cent from France. These unusual percentages reveal that BibSonomy is a local tool strongly established in Germany but with little international impact. This is confirmed by the Country Spreading indicator that shows that close to 74 per cent of users are concentrated in the first ten countries.

Figure 3.7 presents the distribution of users by the year in which they posted their last item. This allows us to observe the evolution of the activity according to the posting performance of the users. The trend shows that the posting performance increases until 2008 in the case of bookmarks and until 2009 regarding publications. The columns then fall until 2013, when there is slight upturn that is more visible in publications. This distribution indicates that there is a standstill during the period 2009–12, brought about perhaps by users leaving, while the peak in 2014 would correspond to active members. Even so, 21 per cent of active users have posted material after 2014, which shows that the network is maintaining a certain amount of activity and still displays updated resources. This would seem to contradict the fall in items posted seen earlier in Figure 3.6, where the number of documents posted has fallen since 2011. This is

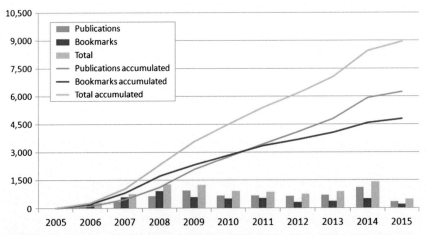

Figure 3.7 Number of members by year in which the last paper was posted in BibSonomy.

explained by the fact that the site has lost a large number of users, so the number of items posted has gone down. However, while there are much fewer users than before, the small fraction of those remaining are more active and maintain the site with an acceptable updating service.

3.2.3 Social Dimension

One of the objectives of any social bookmarking tool is to create a collaborative environment in which members can interact among themselves, sharing their posted documents and organizing their libraries with tags in common. This implies that in spite of posting and tagging being personal actions to address a private benefit, they are also public and can be reutilized by other members. Although no direct collaborative actions are supported, BibSonomy does facilitate several tools to reinforce interaction between members. Users can add other users as friends, sharing the bookmarks and following the activities of others. However, these actions are not public and it is not possible to know who is a friend of whom, which could indicate the degree of involvement in the network.

Another possibility for interaction is to discuss and comment on the literature uploaded by other members. Users can include comments on any post as well as rate it according its value. These comments and ratings are visible to the entire community, encouraging the discussion on the content of new items and ranking documents by the punctuations received.

3.2.3.1 The BibSonomy's Meeting Point

The main collaborative tool in BibSonomy is Groups, where it is possible to create a private environment and where group of members can post each other websites or bibliographies for a particular purpose. For example, a group may be created to post information that is only visible to a specific public. In order to avoid spammers, BibSonomy only permits the setting up of groups after the permission of the administrator has been requested. With regard to authorization, the rest of the members have to ask the creator of the group to be included. These draconian measures would explain the scarce proliferation of groups in this service. In a search by crawler performed in April 2015, 332 groups were identified, a figure that seems rather small for a community of 8,947 active users. In fact, these groups include 1,615 (18 per cent) users, a percentage somewhat higher than that observed in CiteULike but in line with the poor participation in these common spaces. On average, these groups number six users and only 219 (65 per cent) of the groups have more than two members. These groups are close to the size of a workgroup, in which a small number of people employ this function to gather shared resources. In spite of the restrictive criteria to avoid spammers, 52 groups (15 per cent) did not develop any activity, with no bookmarks or publications posted.

Table 3.6 presents the ten most relevant groups ranked by rate of member posts (activity). In BibSonomy, the number of users by group is more balanced although the average activity in the groups (189.8) is much higher than CiteULike, demonstrating that BibSonomy's groups have very high energy. In terms of bookmarks and publications, there are on average almost the double the number of bookmarks (1,032) than publications (626) posted to these groups. This differs from the global data, where the proportion of publications is higher than bookmarks. This could be due in great part to the publications in the general database automatically coming from the DBLP, while groups only include resources manually introduced by their members. This, perhaps, suggests that users' groups prefer to post web resources which are more ephemeral and volatile than publications and therefore it is necessary to conserve their links before being deleted or moved.

The names of the most active groups suggest that many specialize in Computer and Information Sciences. For instead, the *Knowledge and Data Engineering Group* and *bibsonomy_dev* are two examples of groups specializing in computing research. These names also illustrate the different reasons for the creation of a group in a bookmarking service. For example, there are many sites that belong to the research groups, the *Knowledge and Data Engineering Group* and the *Data Mining and Information Retrieval Group (University Würzburg)*, which employ this functionality to organize and create an updated library of bibliographic resources important for their studies. Other groups are related to the research project, the *Tagora Project*, which utilise this service to gather web and bibliographic resources to document their tasks. Other utilities support conferences (*15th Discovery Challenge*) or teaching classes (*uw_ss15_web2.0*). This wide typology of groups is clear evidence of the heterogeneous uses to which this functionality can be put.

It is interesting to note that many of the most active groups have been set up by the same users who participate in several groups at same time, for example: *@hotho* is part of 23 groups, included the ten most active; *@dbenz* posts resources to the *Tagora Project*, the *Tagging Survey*, the *LinkingLinke-Group* and the *Knowledge and Data Engineering Group*;

Table 3.6 The ten groups with the highest activity in BibSonomy in April 2015

Group	Name	Bookmarks	Publications	Total posts	Members	Activity
taggingsurvey	Tagging Survey	5,197	2,676	7,873	11	715.7
linkinglinke	LinkingLinke-Group	4,077	1,587	5,664	10	566.4
bibsonomy_dev	bibsonomy_dev	7,924	3,717	11,641	21	554.3
20dc13	15th Discovery Challenge	5,041	3,176	8,217	15	547.8
Tagora	Tagora Project	9,685	5,536	15,221	28	543.6
uw_ss15_web2.0	uw_ss15_web2.0	4,501	1,930	6,431	13	494.7
Kde	Knowledge and Data Engineering Group	11,291	7,604	18,895	39	484.5
Mykde	Mykde	3,128	2,517	5,645	12	470.4
Sensinthecity	Sensinthecity Project	4,847	2,546	7,393	17	434.9
Dmir	Data Mining and Information Retrieval Group (University Würzburg)	4,501	1,941	6,442	15	429.5
Total		206,416	170,373	376,789	1,675	380.4
Average		1,032.08	626.37	1,308.29	5.98	189.8

and @*stumme* collaborates in the *Tagora Project*, the *Knowledge and Data Engineering Group*, the *Sensinthecity Project* and *Mykde* as well. This would be surprising were it not that they are the creators of the project. This suggests that most of the activities of these groups is performed by members of the research groups that developed the project. So, it is possible that the actual performance of this service, excluding the users that manage the site, is lower than that observed.

However, if we observe the group activity from a temporal perspective, we can see that most of the BibSonomy groups are very active (see Figure 3.8). Of these groups 46 per cent have posted some resource since 2014, being 2015 the year in which the most groups posted documents (35 per cent). In addition, more of the half of the documents had been posted to these groups before 2012 (55 per cent). This behaviour is similar to that observed in the general posting activity, which also shows high levels of recent posting. Therefore BibSonomy shows that, in spite of there being few users on the platform, those users are very active both in profiles and in groups.

3.2.3.2 Tabs, Linking Documents

As on any social bookmarking site, Bibsonomy uses a tagging system to organise, store and retrieve documents posted. These tags are created by the users themselves, although the system has the ability to extract keywords from the text and suggest those terms as tags. Bibsonomy uses a recommendation system adapted from the PageRank algorithm, FolkRank (Benz et al., 2010). In this case, a tag is more important according to the

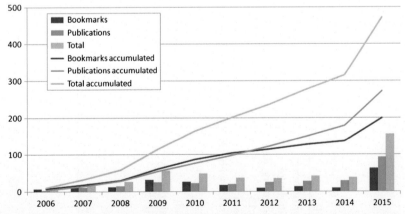

Figure 3.8 Number of groups by year in which the last paper was posted in BibSonomy.

Table 3.7 The ten most used tags in Bibsonomy

Tags	Frequency	%
software	15,590	3.51
Deutschland	12,871	2.90
myown	12,533	2.82
web2.0	10,739	2.42
programming	10,639	2.40
web	10,178	2.29
tolos	9,872	2.22
blog	8,708	1.96
Humans	8,491	1.91
Theorie	8,470	1.91
Total	443,722	100

times that it is used and who uses it. For example, tags used very frequently in the system and inserted by very active users are more relevant than tags infrequently from sporadic members. The aim of this rank is to avoid spam and select the hottest terms by common users in the network.

BibSonomy only lists the hundred tags most used by the community, which are assigned to 443,722 documents. Table 3.7 selects the ten most frequent tags in April 2015, reporting that many of the posted documents belong to Computer and Information Sciences, a similar fact already observed in groups. It is thus possible to observe *software*, *web2.0* and *programming* as specific terms linked to computing disciplines. Another interesting fact is the presence of German language keywords (i.e. *Deutschland*, *Theorie*), which would confirm that this service is principally used by scholars from Germany.

However, the use of tags as a knowledge organization system is problematic because these labels are not restricted to any classification scheme and therefore it is not possible to establish hierarchical relationships between them, ranging from very specific words to keywords with a broad meaning. BibSonomy introduces concepts as a way to solve this limitation. Concepts are terms that group a wide range of tags that belong to the same semantic field. In this way, each concept acts as a generic term that brings together other narrow terms, thus creating hierarchical dependences among tags.

BibSonomy does not make available the full list of concepts, only the fifty most used by the community. Table 3.8 shows the five concepts that most tags group. Two things are evident in this list. The first is that

Table 3.8 The five concepts with the most tags in BibSonomy

Concepts	Tags
Software	183
computer	128
programming	128
People	121
Web	102

the most used concepts belong to the computing research field such as *software*, *computer* or *programming*, which verifies again that this social network is mainly used by users coming from that scientific area. The other interesting observation is that some of these concepts are rather broad and imprecise, without a clear meaning. For example, *people*, *web* or *research* are very generic concepts that do not allow us to know what tags are under those words. Concepts could be a solution to introduce a certain structure to the tagging process but the results prove that they only reproduce the same problems observed in the folksonomy system and suggest that a more structured classification system is needed.

3.2.4 A Local Project

BibSonomy was born with a clear commitment to Science 2.0 and with the solid belief that folksonomy and social tagging are efficient and original ways of managing knowledge. Thus the entire site is organized by tags, which are the principal instruments for navigating through the service in search of relevant information resources as well as the fundamental feature of the building of a stable community of scholars. This mix between knowledge organization and social collaboration lays the foundation for the emergence of new ways of finding information such as serendipity or browsing. But in addition, BibSonomy explores in depth the chances that offer the different relationships between tags, in order to create new practical notions such as Concepts, which will lead to improvements in the search and management of information. The most original contribution of BibSonomy is the clear distinction between posting web resources and bibliographic references, establishing itself between a classical bookmarking service and an online reference management tool. In this way, it broadens the information sources that feed the system and enriches the possibilities of use.

On the other hand, BibSonomy arose from an academic environment set up by a small number of scholars devoted to web programming and knowledge management in Germany. However, the site has not progressed beyond this foundational space and become a global instrument for the entire scientific community. Thus the most used tags and concepts, as well as the affiliations of profiles, demonstrate that BibSonomy continues to be a local tool used mainly by German-speaking and other European users. One other consequence may be seen in the thematic distribution of tags and concepts, which provide evidence of an almost exclusive presence of content related to the Computer and Information Sciences. In general, BibSonomy demonstrates little growth, a fact not only evidenced by the environment in which it situated, but by the actual size of the site. BibSonomy has only 8,900 active users – very low for an academic social site. However, this becomes even more meaningful when it is highlighted that more than 900,000 users are registered on the website. It is evident that this loss of users indicates a high degree of disaffection with the platform.

However, BibSonomy survives. The activity observed among users and groups shows that there is a high proportion of users (21 per cent) and groups (46 per cent) that keep on posting resources. In this way, although the site has lost a considerable number of users and the rate of documents being posting has fallen, the performance of the site is still good thanks to the current users. As we have seen, many of these active users are the founding members and creators of the site who maintaining a high level of activity both in groups and individually. This could distort the perception of the site a little and it is possible that the figures observed would be worse without the stimulated participation of these founder members.

Finally, an important critique of BibSonomy is the employment of data from the DBLP database. There is no problem in taking data from secondary sources to feed the system as this is usual in other information web resources. However, this could distort the view of the site as these records are not in actual fact posted by an individual but are automatically added by the system. This inflates the perception that the content network is growing thanks to the particular activity of its users when the reality is that 76.9 per cent of publications are not posted by the members at all. In fact the activities of the current diminished number of users alone is not enough to keep the site active with recent and varied posts. In addition, this reveals an important limitation of the social bookmarking model, that these spaces only properly work if there is a large and varied critical mass that energises the platform (de Borchgrave, Sanderson, & Harned, 2007). This finding casts serious doubts about the folksonomy and the possibilities of creating suitable information resources.

3.3 THE SOCIAL BENEFIT OF EGOISM

Social bookmarking sites come as an alternative to the existing scientific information services. From a social perspective, these systems aimed to build bibliographic information systems based on the unselfish attitude of individual scholars towards uploading and tagging records. Following a Smithsonian principle,[1] the egotistical interest of each user in creating and managing his or her own library produces an organized bibliographic system useful for the entire community. This egotistical attitude has been observed in the poor use of collaborative tools. Thus, the percentage of active members participating in groups is 18 per cent in BibSonomy and 13.9 per cent in CiteULike. When other tools are analysed, the situation is even worst. The blogs and forums on CiteULike are not being used at all, and the rating and discussion of posts in BibSonomy is anecdotal (5.8 per cent). These percentages demonstrate that the users of social bookmarking sites are not truly interested in social networking but rather in taking advantage of the resulting system. Du, Chu, Gorman, and Siu (2014), surveying Connotea's users, concluded that most of the members used Connotea for personal information management instead of group purposes. However, although not many users wish to participate in groups, those that do keep the rate of activity higher than the average. Thus, CiteULike's groups post 106 papers on average while for the entire site it is 25.7; in BibSonomy 189.8 items on average are uploaded to groups while 101.3 documents on average are posted by each user. In the case of BibSonomy, the group's activity is not only higher but it is also more up to date. While 46 per cent of groups have posted something since 2014, only 9 per cent of CiteULike's groups added any posts in the same time period. This suggests that BibSonomy is in better health than CiteULike, which has suffered a generalized falling off since 2009.

Thus the successful element in a social bookmarking site is the amount of content that its users contribute to the system, so that the more bibliographic records are tagged and shared, the more valuable is the website as scientific information source. According to this idea, CiteULike jumps ahead of BibSonomy. It is the largest service in number of posted publications (8 million records) and registered users (208,000 users approx.), in contrast to the 3.45 million items and 8,947 active users in BibSonomy. In addition, CiteULike has spread across the web sphere in a uniform way, reaching all disciplines and users from all over the world. Hence, the disciplines with the most users are the Biological Sciences (14 per cent) and Medicine (11 per cent), the research areas that produce most results, while the countries with most users are United States (27 per cent) and United Kingdom (11 per cent), the first two scientific powers. However, BibSonomy seems not to have managed going beyond the local surrounding, remaining a site specializing in Computing and Information Sciences – the most frequent tags and concepts come from that research area – and limited to a German-speaking population (41 per cent).

Both sites, born in 2006, are the most relevant examples of social bookmarking for scientists today. They represent the archetype of the folksonomy and social tagging ideas, creating self-organized information systems where the individual action of each user may produce a complex system of scientific information. The folksonomy dream has resulted in a stagnated space (CiteULike), a local and reduced service (BibSonomy) and other sites that have disappeared altogether (Connotea, Collab2), demonstrating that social bookmarking presents more problems than advantages for information management. However, in spite of not having entirely succeeded as social sites and with low levels of collaboration and interaction among their users, they indeed were pioneers in the building of a collaborative environment for sharing references and tags. While their decline could not have been avoided, new collaborative tools such as reference management occupy their space in the social sharing of scientific resources.

NOTE

1. A. Smith (1776) *An Inquiry into the Nature and Causes of the Wealth of Nations*. London: W. Strahan & T. Cadell.

REFERENCES

Benz, D., Hotho, A., Jäschke, R., Krause, B., Mitzlaff, F., Schmitz, C., et al. (2010). The social bookmark and publication management system BibSonomy. *VLDB Journal*, *19*(6), 849–875.

BibSonomy blog. (2007). Feature of the week: Integration of data from the DBLP server. Available from: <http://blog.bibsonomy.org/2007/06/feature-of-week-integration-of-data.html> 10.09.15.

BibSonomy blog. (2009). Tagging for championship. Available from: <http://blog.bibsonomy.org/2009/09/tagging-for-championship.html> 10.09.15.

Bogers, T., & Van den Bosch, A. (2008). Recommending scientific articles using citeulike: *Proceedings of the 2008 ACM conference on recommender*. New York: ACM.

Borrego, A., & Fry, J. (2012). Measuring researchers' use of scholarly information through social bookmarking data: a case study of BibSonomy. *Journal of Information Science*, *38*(3), 297–308.

de Borchgrave, A., Sanderson, T., & Harned, J. (2007). *Force multiplier for intelligence.* Washington, DC: Centre for Strategic and International Studies.

Du, H. S., Chu, S. K., Gorman, G. E., & Siu, F. L. (2014). Academic social bookmarking: An empirical analysis of Connotea users. *Library and Information Science Research, 36*(1), 49–58.

Emamy, K., & Cameron, R. (2007). Citeulike: A researcher's social bookmarking service. *Ariadne,* 51. Available from: <http://www.ariadne.ac.uk/issue51/emamy-cameron/> 10.09.15.

Gilmour, R., & Cobus-Kuo, L. (2011). Reference management software: A comparative analysis of four products. *Issues in Science and Technology Librarianship, 66*(66), 63–75.

Good, B. M., Tennis, J. T., & Wilkinson, M. D. (2009). Social tagging in the life sciences: Characterizing a new metadata resource for bioinformatics. *BMC Bioinformatics, 10,* 313. Available from: <http://www.biomedcentral.com/1471-2105/10/313> 10.09.15.

Hayman, S. (2007). Folksonomies and tagging: New developments in social bookmarking. In *Ark Group Conference: Developing and Improving Classification Schemes.* Sydney. Available from: <http://www.educationau.edu.au/jahia/webdav/site/myjahiasite/shared/papers/akhayman.pdf> 10.09.15.

HESA. (2015). *Joint Academic Coding System (JACS) Version 3.0.* Available from: <https://www.hesa.ac.uk/jacs3> 10.09.15.

Hotho, A., Jäschke, R., Schmitz, C., & Stumme, G. (2006). Information retrieval in folksonomies: Search and ranking. In Y. Sure & J. Domingue (Eds.), *Proceedings of the 3rd European semantic web conference.* Berlin: Springer.

Jäschke, R., Hotho, A., Schmitz, C., & Stumme, G. (2006). Analysis of the publication sharing behaviour in BibSonomy. In S. Polovina, U. Priss, & R. Hill (Eds.), *Proceedings of the conceptual structures: Knowledge architectures for smart applications.* Berlin: Springer.

Jiang, J., He, D., & Ni, C. (2011). Social reference: Aggregating online usage of scientific articles in CiteULike for clustering academic resources: *ACM/IEEE joint conference on digital libraries.* New York: ACM.

Lee, D.H., & Brusilovsky, P. (2010). Interest similarity of group members: The case study of Citeulike, In *Proceedings of the WebSci10: Extending the Frontiers of Society On-Line.* Raleigh, NC: WebSci. Available from: <http://journal.webscience.org/362/2/websci10_submission_64.pdf> 10.09.15.

Marieke, G., & Tonkin, E. (2006). Folksonomies tidying up tags. *D-Lib Magazine, 12,* 1.

Mathes, A. (2004). Folksonomies – cooperative classification and communication through shared metadata: *Computer-Mediated communication, LIS5900CMC (Doctoral seminar).* University of Illinois Urbana-Champaign, Graduate School of Library and Information Science.

Mendeley blog. (2009). CiteULike and Mendeley collaborate. Available from: <http://blog.mendeley.com/academic-features/citeulike-and-mendeley-collaborate/> 10.09.15.

Santos-Neto, E., Condon, D., Andrade, N., Iamnitchi, A., & Ripeanu, M. (2014). Reuse, temporal dynamics, interest sharing, and collaboration in social tagging systems. *First Monday, 19*(7) Available from: <http://firstmonday.org/ojs/index.php/fm/article/view/4994/4101> 10.09.15.

Wikipedia. (2015). BibSonomy. Available from: <http://en.wikipedia.org/wiki/BibSonomy> 10.09.15.

CHAPTER 4

Reference Management Tools

Software for reference management was born in the early 1980s to support the academic activities of the users, allowing the organization of large bibliographic databases and the use of these references for the elaboration of scholarly documents. ProCite and Reference Manager were the first solutions of this type and they consisted of a system for managing a bibliographic database and several outputs such as bibliographies, citation styles and a gateway to include citations in word processors. However, these products could only be fed manually or through the Z39.50 protocol (Miller, 1993). The Web posed, in this sense, a great opportunity because it made it possible to access a wide range of bibliographic sources and collect many types of items. This change promoted a new generation of reference managers and Mendeley, Zotero, EndNote and RefWorks, for example, emerged as systems that capture bibliographic metadata included in web pages (Norman, 2010). So, it was not surprising that Zotero was born as a Mozilla plug-in that captured references while surfing the Web or that Mendeley relies on data extraction from multiple web sources. In this way, reference management tools moved from the desktop to the Web to increase their bibliographic services as well as enhance their attractiveness with networking functionalities.

However, these applications did not develop in response to a collaborative need, as happened with social bookmarking sites. Reference management tools are products oriented to individual users that aim to have a large bibliographic database that supports their personal scientific activities (writing papers, being informed in their research fields, etc.). Therefore, the functionalities of these systems do not depend on the social involvement of their users, but on individual purposes oriented to make the most of their libraries. Why then have these products developed social networking platforms? The response may be found precisely in the influence of the bookmarking sites and the way in which these sites feed their systems. As it has been seen, social bookmarking platforms were forerunners of these bibliographic services that succeeded thanks to the participative activity of their users putting and tagging information into the system.

Social Network Sites for Scientists.
ISBN 978-0-08-100592-7

It is possible that reference management tools observed this model and they find in users the possibility of increasing their sources with non published materials, data sets and web pages, as well as taking advantage of the document usage for producing statistics on information consumption (i.e. Readers in Mendeley).

Reference management sites could therefore be considered one step more advanced than social bookmarking sites because they take from the latter their main social tools such as tags, groups, followers, etc. and join them to a powerful bibliographic service. In this way, reference management tools transcend personal functions and create a global information system enriched by the social interaction of their users. In other words, reference management systems jump from the individual desktop to the social web and incorporate all the networking instruments already introduced by bookmarking sites. It can be said then that reference management sites are one step further in the evolution of academic social sites because they combine the power of a scientific information system and the flexibility of an open social sharing platform.

This chapter focuses on the two most representative bibliographic management tools that incorporate social networking utilities. Mendeley and Zotero are the only platforms that achieve those requirements as well as being open and freely accessible to any scholar. (This is the reason that EndNote is not analysed in this study, because its social network is only accessible for private customers of Thomson Reuters.)

4.1 MENDELEY

Mendeley is a reference management platform that is set up with two basic elements: desktop software and a social website. The first is a local database management system of bibliographic references and the second is a web platform to share these references. The product was started in 2008 by Jan Reichelt, Victor Henning and Paul Föckler, a group of German scholars specializing in information studies who met in London. The objective of this initiative was to create an application that would enable the management of bibliographic references as well as make it possible to share and discuss these documents with others. For this they were inspired by the music platform Last.fm, from which they took the principal elements (Henning & Reichelt, 2008) of an open database, usage-based metrics and collaborative filtering. Since its release, the site has been honoured with prizes and awards. However, in 2013 it was purchase by

Elsevier, one of the giants of academic publishing. This produced an angry outburst as many users considered Mendeley to be an example of the Open Access movement, and this integration with Elsevier would break its commitment (Anderson, 2013).

4.1.1 Desktop App

The desktop application is software that allows the creation of a database of bibliographic references to be used to generate bibliographies and to manage the citations included in a academic paper. Using a plug-in, this software is connected to any text processor (MS Word, Mac Word, LibreOffice, BibTex), enabling the use of the database to insert citations in the text and generate reference lists. It accepts a large amount of citation styles and also incorporates a CSL editor to enable the design of a personal style (Zaugg, West, Tateishi, & Randall, 2011).

In addition, it incorporates a PDF reader, which when linked to the bibliographic database, makes it possible to manage a full text bibliographic database. In this form, the reader permits the extraction of metadata from each PDF file to be included in the database. In addition, this collection of PDFs is organized as a library, where the full texts of the documents are indexed and therefore can be retrieved using any relevant word. This reader acts as a text editor, which allows the inclusion of notes and the highlighting of relevant sections of the text as well.

Mendeley also acts as a bookmarking service in the same way as CiteULike, BibSonomy or Connotea. Through a plug-in installed in the web browser, bibliographic references can be incorporated from the most important publisher sites and scientific information services. Mendeley accepts multiple importing formats such as BibTeX, RIS and EndNote XML, which means that it directly accepts records from Zotero, Papers and EndNote, their principal competitors. In addition, Mendeley is compatible with any operating system and offers access from the Web, smartphones and any other device.

4.1.2 The Crowdsourced Catalogue

Mendeley maintains a public bibliographic database from the records inserted by each user in his/her private personal library. Hence, whenever users upload references to My Publications, these appear in the global web collection of Mendeley, the rest remaining hidden on the desktops of the users. In May 2015 Mendeley made the extravagant claim of more than 500 million papers (CrunchBase, 2015), but this unlikely amount is no doubt the result of the aggregation of every personal library without distinguishing duplicate records. Thus the most up-to-date approximation of the total number of unique papers is 114 million (Pimasoli, 2014). However, it is very hard to work out the real coverage of Mendeley because there are several difficulties in its API in order to retrieve bibliographic data (Gunn, 2013). Moreover, from 2014 the API has not offered any statistical information on the document catalogue, profiles or disciplines. Another limit is the ineffective management of duplicates which could overestimate the real size of the catalogue (Hull, 2010).

In order to remedy this problem, a sample of documents was extracted from Mendeley to analyse the properties of their documents and their origin. In this way, several neutral and broad queries (i.e. *a, the, and*) were launched. English terms were used because this is the principal communication language in Science and these terms would retrieve the largest sample possible. In total, 902,659 documents were extracted from Mendeley's public catalogue.

In addition to the items uploaded by the users, Mendeley extracts bibliographic data from other important sources. Table 4.1 presents the ten most relevant sources that feed into this database. Only 1.7 per cent of documents have no sources, which it could correspond to materials supplied by individual users or sources without publisher. The principal sources for the catalogue are PubMed (18 per cent), Scopus (1.2 per cent) and ScienceDirect (0.6 per cent). The first is a bibliographic database specializing in biomedical documents and the last a citation index and web publishing platform, products owned by Elsevier. This could be due to the

Table 4.1 The ten most important sources in Mendeley

Source	Documents	Documents %
PubMed (www.ncbi.nlm.nih.gov)	162,399	17.99
Scopus (www.scopus.com)	10,699	1.18
ScienceDirect (www.sciencedirect.com)	5,146	0.57
ProQuest (search.proquest.com)	4,795	0.53
Physical Review Letters	3,666	0.41
arXiv.org (*arxiv.org*)	3,607	0.4
Applied optics	3,554	0.4
JSTOR (www.jstor.org)	3,439	0.38
Tetrahedron Letters	2,310	0.25
Optics Letters	2,152	0.24
Total	902,659	100

agreement between Mendeley and Elsevier, according to which the publishing giant contributes references to the Mendeley catalogue. The rest are repositories (ArXiv.org, JSTOR) and specialized databases (ProQuest). This proportion of external sources coincides with the results reported by Hammerton, Granitzer, Harvey, Hristakeva, and Jack (2012).

With regard to the type of document, Mendeley defines several document types according to the fields that each record contains. For example, the number and type of fields for a thesis are different to those of a journal article. Thus Table 4.2 shows the principal document types. The first three – *journal, generic* and *journal article* – correspond to the common journal article, summing up 85 per cent of the type of documents in Mendeley's catalogue. The rest of the materials have a low presence though it is just worth commenting on *Conference Proceedings* (6.1 per cent). These results show the hegemony of the journal articles and the marginal existence of the other formats in the current scientific publishing world.

Mendeley's crowdsourced catalogue is organized around 25 research disciplines and 473 subdisciplines. This classification scheme represents a conceptual structure that not only serves to organize the bibliographic references, but is present in the arrangement of groups and profiles as well. These subject classes come from the Online Computer Library Center

Table 4.2 Catalogue items distributed according to type of document in Mendeley

Type	Documents	% documents
Journal	582,494	64.77
Generic	121,526	13.51
Journal Article	62,602	6.96
Conference Proceedings	55,185	6.14
Case	42,265	4.70
book_section	12,551	1.40
Book	5,152	0.57
Report	4,176	0.46
Thesis	3,622	0.40
Newspaper Article	2,907	0.32
Patent	2,786	0.31
Magazine Article	1,880	0.21
WebPage	1,414	0.16
working_paper	463	0.05
Bill	173	0.02
EncyclopediaArticle	133	0.01
Total	899,329	100

(OCLC), a consortium of libraries assembled to reduce costs and improve access to information.

Mendeley uses a peculiar criterion to assign papers to these subject classes. This process is made according to the readers of the documents. Thus a paper is not assigned to a discipline by its content, but by who its readers are. In this way a paper is classified as Mathematics if the highest percentage of its readers come from a Mathematics background. This would be correct if the paper had a large number of readers as it is logical that users would be interested in papers from their own research area. But for the majority of papers which barely reach ten readers (85 per cent), this criterion would produce a certain randomness and generate a serious problem of misclassification. This could mean, for example, that a paper published in a mathematics journal and tagged with mathematics keywords is assigned to Physics because a physicist user decided to include that reference in his or her library. Thus classification is influenced by the readers' field of study, so as many users from a discipline read a paper more likely that paper is assigned to that disciplinary group. It is not surprising therefore that the thematic distribution of papers coincides with the distribution of users, as will be seen later. To avoid this limitation and increase the findability, Mendeley also links each document with the other two most frequent disciplines of their readers. For example, a paper assigned to Mathematics could be retrieved by Physics and Computer and Information Science as well due to the second and third group of readers belong to those disciplines.

Figure 4.1 and Table 4.3 show the percentage of retrieved, assigned and open papers by discipline, that is records that can be searched in the Papers section. Retrieving documents by discipline, the aggregated total is 66.2 million. As we saw above, this number is arrived at because the same paper can be linked to up to three disciplines. Taking only the principal discipline, the total number of uploaded papers by the users to the public catalogue is 14.7 million documents, a percentage rather low according to the global estimate of 114 million in the system (Pimasoli, 2014). This could indicate that approximately nine out ten documents are privately managed in each user's library, a figure that is not very optimistic for the sharing of documents in Mendeley.

According to assigned papers, the research areas with highest representation are *Biological Sciences* (23.8 per cent), *Medicine* (14.5 per cent) and *Engineering* (7.2 per cent). These proportions are a little different according to open papers. Thus *Medicine* contains 22.5 per cent of open documents,

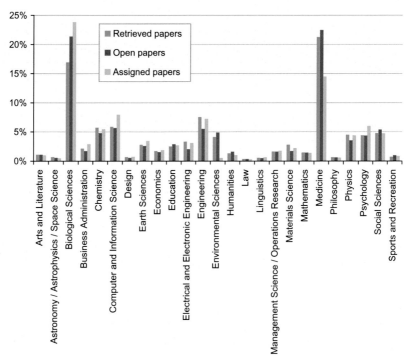

Figure 4.1 Number of retrieved papers, assigned papers and open papers by research discipline in Mendeley.

Biological Sciences 21.4 per cent and *Computer and Information Science* 5.7 per cent. In total, only 3.1 million articles (4.7 per cent) are open access. However, this definition only includes articles published in open journals. Mendeley allows authors to deposit a full-text copy of any paper in their personal profile, which is accessible to registered users only. Therefore, if these copies were considered 'open', the proportion of open articles would be higher. In any case, regarding to the rate of open/not open articles per discipline, *Sports and Recreation* (6.3 per cent) show the highest proportion, followed by *Biological Sciences* (5.9 per cent) and *Humanities* (5.6 per cent), whereas *Electrical and Electronic Engineering* (2.9 per cent) and *Materials Science* (2.9 per cent) are the disciplines with less open papers.

Mendeley introduces an original indicator to measure the quality of a paper in its catalogue. 'Readers' is the number of times that a document has been included in a personal library (Gunn, 2013). In this way, Mendeley assumes that if a paper is referenced in a personal library then it could mean that the paper is valuable for that user. Thus, as more papers

Table 4.3 Distribution of papers and open papers by discipline in Mendeley

Discipline	Retrieved papers	% retrieved papers	Assigned papers	% assigned papers	Open papers	% open papers	Open ratio %
Arts and Literature	740,576	1.12	148,902	1.01	34,558	1.11	4.67
Astronomy/Astrophysics/ Space Science	464,153	0.70	74,511	0.50	17,413	0.56	3.75
Biological Sciences	11,220,236	16.95	3522,515	23.84	663,696	21.38	5.92
Business Administration	1,430,541	2.16	431,770	2.92	53,615	1.73	3.75
Chemistry	3,795,153	5.73	807,677	5.47	148,844	4.79	3.92
Computer and Information Science	3,895,713	5.88	1180,377	7.99	176,015	5.67	4.52
Design	464,982	0.70	110,229	0.75	17,349	0.56	3.73
Earth Sciences	1,867,589	2.82	512,748	3.47	80,798	2.60	4.33
Economics	1,146,552	1.73	280,521	1.90	48,207	1.55	4.20
Education	1,670,102	2.52	398,967	2.70	89,898	2.90	5.38
Electrical and Electronic Engineering	2,212,595	3.34	459,164	3.11	63,513	2.05	2.87
Engineering	5,019,852	7.58	1,070,536	7.24	171,058	5.51	3.41
Environmental Sciences	2,734,764	4.13	79,649	0.54	151,809	4.89	5.55
Humanities	888,296	1.34	154,245	1.04	50,129	1.61	5.64
Law	246,379	0.37	44,579	0.30	11,575	0.37	4.70
Linguistics	379,322	0.57	99,724	0.67	15,977	0.51	4.21
Management Science / Operations Research	1,087,499	1.64	263,046	1.78	50,509	1.63	4.64
Materials Science	1,865,872	2.82	328,969	2.23	53,416	1.72	2.86
Mathematics	971,295	1.47	206,470	1.40	45,183	1.46	4.65
Medicine	14,095,009	21.29	2,141,119	14.49	698,024	22.48	4.95
Philosophy	444,741	0.67	90,125	0.61	19,352	0.62	4.35
Physics	2,980,905	4.50	649,394	4.39	110,038	3.54	3.69
Psychology	2,921,248	4.41	889,509	6.02	135,438	4.36	4.64
Social Sciences	3,164,958	4.78	703,412	4.76	167,333	5.39	5.29
Sports and Recreation	491,665	0.74	128,317	0.87	31,182	1.00	6.34
Total	66,199,997	100	14,776,475	100	3,104,929	100	4.69

are used in a personal library, the higher the quality and the more appreciated they are by the scholarly community. However, this assumption cannot be related to citation impact, firstly because a paper included in a library does not directly mean that it has been read, and secondly, the inclusion of a paper in a library is not always motivated by impact or quality reasons (Mohammadi, Thelwall, & Kousha, 2015a). Another problem is that the population distribution affects the readership of papers. Thus a paper is more likely to be read by a numerous type of user (e.g. students, Americans, etc.) than by other groups. Even so, this statistic is a good indicator of the use of these documents by the members' network, supplying information on the status, discipline and location of their readers.

Apart from the meaning of this index, Figure 4.2 plots the power law distribution of the number of readers by research paper. From the sample 190,559 (21 per cent) papers do not have any reader or their readers 'are being calculated'. This figure shows a markedly skewed distribution ($\gamma = 3.49$) where a very large proportion of papers is read by just one or two users. In fact, half of the papers have less than two readers and 85 per cent have less than ten, with an average of 5.4 readers per document. These results show that most of the papers pass unnoticed by the scholarly community and only a small fraction of papers causes any impact in the population in terms of readership.

However, this fact raises some doubts about the disciplinary classification of documents. As has been seen, half of papers are read by less than two users, which means that half of the papers are classified only by the

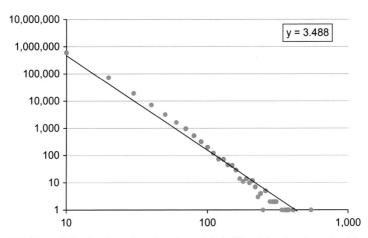

Figure 4.2 Binned distribution of readers by article in Mendeley (log-log plot; bin = 10).

subjective opinion of one or two users. This can produce a very random assignation procedure and is an important weakness in the classification system.

4.1.3 The Social Network

The structural participation framework of Mendeley is set up by three key elements: individual users through profiles, collective users through groups, and the tags as instrument of information organization.

4.1.3.1 Tags or Keywords?

It could be said that tags are reminiscent of the social bookmarking sites, where they were key elements in the thematic structuring of content. From a certain viewpoint, they represent traces of the several loans that Mendeley makes from previous academic social sites to configure its web service. However, the role of tags in Mendeley is not so important as in CiteUlike and BibSonomy. In Mendeley, documents are classified beforehand following a structural scheme, and the tags are used simply as navigational tools that broaden the retrieval possibilities of the system. In addition, many of these tags are automatically added from the author's keywords, so analysis of these labels would result in confusion as it is not easy to distinguish between users' tags and authors' keywords. A recent analysis found 6.13 tags per document with a median of 3 in computer science articles (Pimasoli, 2014). These results describe an elevated ratio of tags, despite the majority of them being supplied by the author him or herself.

4.1.3.2 Profiles, the Students' Network

Besides being a reference management tool, Mendeley also acts as a document sharing site. This means that each user can upload their own publications to be read and downloaded by the rest of members. However, this functionality causes some confusion because many users consider that section to be a personal library as well, and they post no authored papers. It is not possible to know how often this is the case, but it could influence further comparisons with other document sharing sites. Each profile contains identification data such as affiliation, location and discipline. This last is mandatory when a profile is created, as well as the academic position. In addition, the profile shows several statistics that describe the performance of the profile in the network. Thus the number of publications is the number of documents uploaded to the profile, while 'Readers'

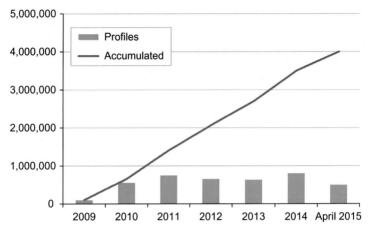

Figure 4.3 Evolution of number of profiles in Mendeley.

refers the number of users that have included some paper from that profile in their libraries. Other indicators (followers/followings) describe social interactions with other users following the updates of their profiles with new papers and other activities. Each profile is informed of this activity through a Dashboard, where he or she is alerted to the recent activity of their followers and groups.

Figure 4.3 shows the evolution of the number of users in Mendeley since 2009. The WayBack Machine of Archive.org and the Mendeley blog were used to extract the more approximate figures. The addition of users to Mendeley follows a linear trend with an average annual growth (CAGR = 63 per cent) since 2009. The incorporation of new profiles is similar each year, while the addition of new users following a pause in the rate may be noted, and the 2011–13 period shows a mild deceleration. In this sense, although Mendeley increases its members each year, the rate is rather slow and this could be due to signs of exhaustion.

A more detailed analysis of Mendeley's profiles was carried out to study the disciplinary, geographic, institutional and academic post distribution of its users. Mendeley has a search interface to find other colleagues and follow them. However, this mechanism is rather rudimentary and only retrieves profiles with an exact match and is lacking in wildcards or other types of operators. In addition, it only indexes the names of the profiles, so it is not possible to obtain profiles by affiliation, location, discipline, etc. Thus, to extract a representative and random sample of profiles, more than 3,000 of the most frequent names in the world were selected to query the

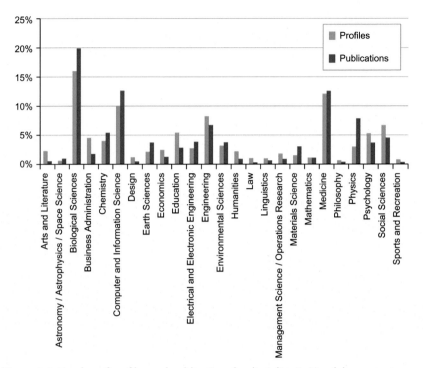

Figure 4.4 Number of profiles and publications by discipline in Mendeley.

system. In total, 1,029,998 profiles were retrieved from Mendeley in May 2015, a very large sample that could well be a quarter of the total number of profiles created in the system (four million approximately) (Mendeley blog, 2015).

From a disciplinary view, the distribution of profiles and their publication in Mendeley is quite similar to the distribution of papers and groups. This brings together the document coverage and the users' population and suggests that the taking up of these sites is affected by the contents that are generated in them. Figure 4.4 shows that the network is mainly populated by users from *Biological Sciences* (16 per cent), *Medicine* (12 per cent) and *Computer and Information Science* (10 per cent), a distribution very similar to the distribution of papers in the catalogue. According to the publications of these profiles, *Biological Sciences* (20 per cent) is still the research area that posts most papers, followed by *Medicine* (13 per cent) and *Computer and Information Science* (13 per cent). This is influenced by the number of profiles, which determines the number of publications. However, the rate of publications per profile presents a different figure. Now, it is *Physics*

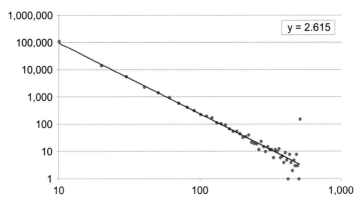

Figure 4.5 Binned distribution of publications by user in Mendeley (log-log plot; bin = 10).

(2.69) that is the discipline posting the most publications host, along with *Material Science* (2.05) and *Earth Sciences* (1.8). This proportion is closer to the usual average of papers by disciplines observed in other academic social sites (Ortega, 2015) and scientific databases (Ioannidis, Boyack, & Klavans, 2014; Ruiz-Castillo and Costas, 2014).

From the sample, only 141,895 (13.7 per cent) users include publications in their profiles, which demonstrates that the possibility to share documents in Mendeley is not entirely utilized by all users. As was said above, Mendeley is somewhat confusing according to the publications that are listed in the profiles, because some users include not authored papers by themselves, thinking that it is an extension of their personal library. Figure 4.5 plots the number of users against the number of papers. The distribution shows a skewed trend ($\gamma = 2.61$) in which a large proportion of users publish a small number of papers, while only a small group of members post a large number of publications. Thus, only 20 per cent of users upload more than ten papers and just 152 profiles post 500 papers, the limit for uploading papers in each profile. The average number of papers is 24.9 per user.

Similar behaviour describes the distribution of followers by profiles, although the exponent ($\gamma = 3.33$) in this case is more pronounced (see Figure 4.6). This means that the imbalance in the number of followers is even more so among the users of Mendeley. Thus 692,275 (67 per cent) profiles do not have any followers and from those remaining, 94 per cent have less than ten followers. However, only two profiles have more than 1,000 followers. The average of followers in Mendeley is around 1. This indicator of social networking informs us that the Mendeley network is

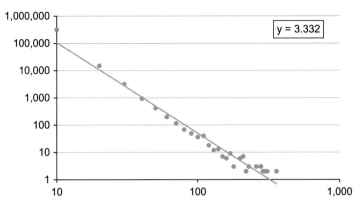

Figure 4.6 Binned distribution of followers by user in Mendeley (log-log plot; bin = 10).

still sparse and only a small number of users are following the careers of other members. This could be due to several facts. The first is that this tool was only recently introduced (Mendeley blog, 2014), and it is possible that many users are not yet using this method of detecting profile updates. Another reason could be related to the availability of this site as a document sharing service and, as has been seen before, this function is not widely used. Therefore, if there are many profiles with no papers or with just a couple, it is logical to conclude that most of the users do not use it to follow other profiles in the network.

Mendeley also makes it compulsory to enter the academic status of its users. Although this information is not present in the profiles, it is indeed visible in the page results when profiles are searched. Following the procedure above, 1.6 million academic statuses were collected from the retrieved profiles. Figure 4.7 shows the distribution of profiles by academic status. The most frequent categories are *Student (Bachelor)* (21.1 per cent), *Student (Master)* (20.7 per cent) and *Ph.D. Student* (15.7 per cent). It is evident that Mendeley is mainly taken up by students (57.5 per cent) that are starting their academic careers. Many of them are involved in doctoral dissertations which demand bibliographic tools such as Mendeley to obtain in-depth knowledge of the current literature in their respective research areas. This distribution, biased towards young and starting scholars, could affect the 'Readers' indicator, as noted above. In this way, the likelihood that a paper is read by a student is more than 50 per cent, so it is not surprising that this type of scholar is reading the most documents in Mendeley (Mohammadi, Thelwall, Haustein, & Larivière, 2015b) and that this platform is preferred by students (Jordan, 2014).

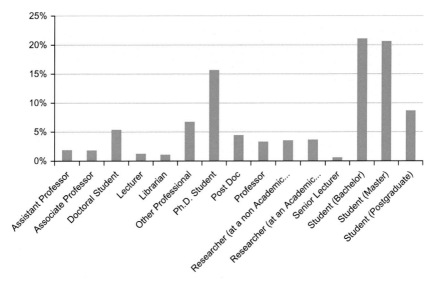

Figure 4.7 Number of profiles by academic status in Mendeley.

From the sample, only 85,713 (8 per cent) users included their affiliation in their profiles, so the institutional representation could be biased and not representative of the entire population in Mendeley. Even so, the organizations with the most profiles are the *Universidade de São Paulo* (0.56 per cent), the *Universidad Nacional Autónoma de México* (0.45 per cent) and the *University of Cambridge* (0.41 per cent), that is large universities in terms of the number of academic staff (see Table 4.4). It is also interesting to note that among the first ten institutions there are four British universities so it is possible that this service, which is headquartered in London, is preferred by British academics. According to the number of publications, the French *CNRS* (0.44 per cent) and the British *University of Oxford* (0.21 per cent) and *University of Cambridge* (0.2 per cent) are the institutions with the most papers posted in Mendeley.

Exploring the distribution by country, 144,721 (14 per cent) users included location in their profiles, a proportion rather high in comparison with sites analysed previously (see Table 4.5). Nevertheless, this proportion casts serious doubt on the readers' statistics at country level as they may not be representative enough (Haunschild, Bornmann, & Leydesdorff, 2015). The countries with the most profiles in the network are the *United States* (22.5 per cent), followed far behind by the *United Kingdom* (9.7 per cent) and *Brazil* (6.7 per cent). With regard to publications, the *United*

Table 4.4 The ten organizations with the most users in Mendeley

Affiliation	Profiles	Profiles %	Publications	Publications %
Universidade de São Paulo	477	0.56	1,782	0.17
Universidad Nacional Autónoma de México	384	0.45	1,746	0.17
University of Cambridge	350	0.41	2,097	0.20
Imperial College London	318	0.37	1,485	0.14
Stanford University	297	0.35	1,110	0.11
University of Oxford	291	0.34	2,256	0.21
Harvard University	290	0.34	1,509	0.14
University of Edinburgh	239	0.28	872	0.08
CNRS	236	0.28	4,639	0.44
Pennsylvania State University	220	0.26	646	0.06
Total	85,713		1,055,752	100

Table 4.5 The ten countries with the most users and publications in Mendeley

Country	Profiles	% profiles	Publications	% publications	Penetration
United States	32,502	22.46	98,886	9.37	1.21
United Kingdom	14,099	9.74	53,322	5.05	2.62
Brazil*	9,725	6.72	24,715	2.34	3.27
Germany	8,987	6.21	35,944	3.40	1.24
Spain	6,931	4.79	39,604	3.75	2.48
Canada	5,331	3.68	17,079	1.62	1.58
France	3,840	2.65	26,950	2.55	0.72
Portugal	3,526	2.44	9,490	0.90	3.29
India*	3,421	2.36	8,246	0.78	0.83
Mexico	3,276	2.26	6,425	0.61	3.31
Total	144,721	100	1,055,752	100	

*2010.

States (9.4 per cent) and the *United Kingdom* (5.1 per cent) are still the countries with highest number of contributions, followed by *Spain* (3.8 per cent) and *Germany* (3.4 per cent). According to the degree of penetration, *Mexico* (3.3) and the two principal Portuguese speaking countries, *Portugal* (3.3) and *Brazil* (3.3), are the countries where Mendeley is most successful, followed by the *United Kingdom* (2.6), the country where this platform is located. The Country Spreading, the percentage of users among the first ten countries, is 63 per cent, the lowest percentage of the sites analysed and shows that this service has reached global diffusion.

4.1.3.3 Groups, the Readers' Club

The third instrument of social participation in Mendeley is groups. These aim to gather together different users to compile specific bibliographies on determined issues or to gather working materials for projects or research groups. In addition to adding references, members' groups can also discuss, rate and comment on these references or another issue.

Table 4.6 and Figure 4.8 show the distribution of groups and the number of papers included in these groups by research discipline. In April 2015, Mendeley counted 97,857 (138,387 by discipline) public groups that might be assigned to several disciplines. The private groups are only visible to their members, so the number of private groups is unknown. Since 2011, the growth of groups has been exponential, with an annual increase of CAGR = 74 per cent (Jeng, He, Jiang, & Zhang, 2012). The thematic distribution of public groups is similar to the number of documents in the public catalogue. Thus the disciplines with the most groups are *Biological Sciences* (17.3 per cent), *Medicine* (12.9 per cent) and *Computer and Information Science* (12.7 per cent). According to the number of papers, 4.6 (5.7 by discipline) million documents were posted to these groups. This means that 31.3 per cent of the papers in the catalogue were shared in groups, which is an appreciable amount. No disciplinary differences exist when it comes to posting papers to the groups, so *Biological Sciences* (23.6 per cent) is the discipline with most posted papers, followed by *Medicine* (12.8 per cent) and *Computer and Information Science* (9.7 per cent). However, there are indeed differences in papers by group rate. The most active disciplines uploading papers are *Environmental Sciences* (60.1 papers by group), *Linguistics* (59.5 papers by group) and *Biological Sciences* (56.5 papers by group). Finally, the number of members that joined up to a group is 275,266, approximately 6.8 per cent of the global community of users (Mendeley blog, 2015), a proportion a little above the 5.7 per cent found by Oh and Jeng (2011). This proportion of users interested in groups is the lowest percentage observed and shows that this functionality is not attractive for most of the users.

If we look at the characteristics of the groups themselves, Table 4.7 shows the ten most active groups. An average of 73 papers is included

Table 4.6 Distribution of groups, members joined and papers posted to groups by research discipline in Mendeley

Disciplines	Groups	Groups %	Papers	Papers %	Papers/group	Members	Activity
Arts and Literature	1,848	1.34	67,855	1.18	36.7	6,718	10.10
Astronomy/Astrophysics/Space Science	776	0.56	23,128	0.40	29.8	2,005	11.54
Biological Sciences	23,955	17.31	1,352,650	23.59	56.5	57,814	23.40
Business Administration	5,060	3.66	98,970	1.73	19.6	16,334	6.06
Chemistry	5,740	4.15	222,369	3.88	38.7	13,698	16.23
Computer and Information Science	17,574	12.70	556,270	9.70	31.7	58,100	9.57
Design	1,734	1.25	46,001	0.80	26.5	6,769	6.80
Earth Sciences	3,143	2.27	174,742	3.05	55.6	9,908	17.64
Economics	3,122	2.26	37,565	0.66	12.0	6,485	5.79
Education	7,015	5.07	204,946	3.57	29.2	27,145	7.55
Electrical and Electronic Engineering	3,746	2.71	132,691	2.31	35.4	8,568	15.49
Engineering	11,849	8.56	368,304	6.42	31.1	24,273	15.17
Environmental Sciences	5,126	3.70	308,137	5.37	60.1	19,448	15.84
Humanities	2,430	1.76	118,346	2.06	48.7	10,337	11.45
Law	764	0.55	20,634	0.36	27.0	2,848	7.25
Linguistics	927	0.67	55,150	0.96	59.5	4,591	12.01
Management Science/Operations Research	2,255	1.63	104,594	1.82	46.4	11,194	9.34
Materials Science	2,542	1.84	114,878	2.00	45.2	6,769	16.97
Mathematics	1,294	0.94	47,455	0.83	36.7	7,440	6.38
Medicine	17,842	12.89	735,583	12.83	41.2	34,423	21.37
Philosophy	728	0.53	28,791	0.50	39.5	4,969	5.79
Physics	4,348	3.14	164,702	2.87	37.9	11,974	13.75
Psychology	7,358	5.32	269,886	4.71	36.7	21,119	12.78
Social Sciences	9,134	6.60	443,652	7.74	48.6	42,128	10.53
Sports and Recreation	1,147	0.83	37,491	0.65	32.7	2,865	13.09
Total	138,387	100	5,734,790	100	40.5	417,922	13.72

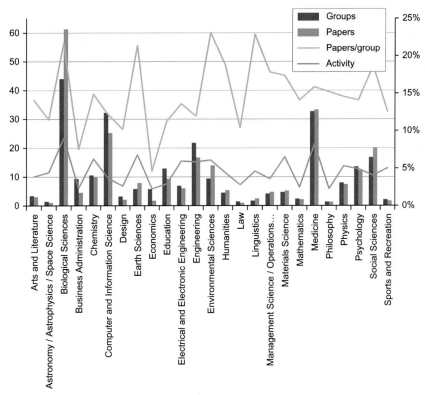

Figure 4.8 Percentage of groups and papers posted to groups by research discipline in Mendeley.

Table 4.7 The ten most active groups in Mendeley

Group	Papers	Members	Activity
Zootaxa	10,902	86	126.77
Public Health England Obesity Knowledge and Intelligence – Knowledge Update	6,326	50	126.52
Amphibian Species of the World	9,556	79	120.96
Traductores e interpretes	5,714	71	80.48
Ecological Anthropology	7,019	128	54.84
Ocean Acidification (OA-ICC)	2,471	51	48.45
New Interfaces for Musical Expression	2,281	59	38.66
POLYMER_BASED NANOCOMPOSITES	2,630	74	35.54
European Journal of Entomology	1,447	50	28.94
Translation Studies	6,336	250	25.34
Total	4,597,979	190,935	8.20
Average	73.02	3.09	26.27

in each set, a rate lower than that observed in CiteUlike (106.3) and BibSonomy (87.3). In addition, the number of members by group (3.1) is rather low, being more than half of the groups (52 per cent) formed by only one member. These values are lower than the figures found by Oh and Jeng (2011), which suggests that participation in groups could increase with time. All these indicators lead us to think that the use of public groups in order to share references is not very frequent and would not attract the attention of many users. As with the case of social bookmarking tools, the typology of groups in Mendeley is quite varied and among the most active groups can be found journal sites (i.e. *Zootaxa*, the *European Journal of Entomology*) that upload their publications to be discussed and read by their members, projects that attempt to create a comprehensive database of references on a specific theme (i.e. *Ocean Acidification (OA-ICC)*, *Amphibian Species of the World*) or simply places where the most recent updates and news on a research line may be found (i.e. *Translation Studies, POLYMER_BASED NANOCOMPOSITES*).

Figure 4.9 allows us to observe the evolution of the activity of these groups over the years. The accumulated line describes an ascending linear trend while the bars reveal a pause in growth. Only 38 per cent of the groups have developed some activity (i.e. posting a paper, inserting a comment) since 2014. This growing pattern provides evidences that although the number of groups is small and the activity is not much higher, a considerable proportion of groups do have a current activity. However, this does not hide the fact that 62 per cent of the groups are losing activity and freshness.

4.1.4 Discovering Recommended Papers

Mendeley is the most well known of the current reference management services due to its success in terms of the number of users – more than four million in 2015 – and, above all, the way in which it has been able to combine a management service of scientific literature with a social network. One of the key strengths of this service is the large and complete database of public bibliographic references, with more than 14 million items available for any user. This fact is not only important in meeting the demands of Mendeley's users, but it also turns it into an important information service comparable to any academic search engine or document sharing system. One might say that Mendeley could become a complete academic site because it is offering several services on the same platform. In this sense, Mendeley has developed from reference management

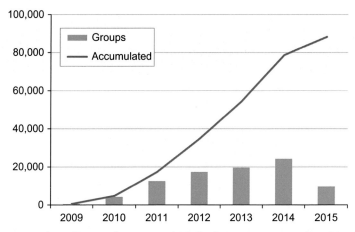

Figure 4.9 Number of groups by year in which the last action was made in Mendeley.

software to become a social bookmarking site with document sharing possibilities and a searchable bibliographic database.

However, this strategy is not giving the expected results in many respects. Mendeley's social network is sparse and weak in comparison with other sites that have been analysed. The average of followers (1.1) points out that the connectivity between users at the individual level is very small and the linear annual growth rate (CAGR = 63 per cent) of new users also evidences a slowing down of Mendeley's community. On the other hand, the percentages involved in filling out profile information (>14 per cent) and the interest in uploading papers (13.7 per cent) give evidence that many users are not registered in Mendeley to share articles or establish personal contacts. Similar underperforming values were observed with regard to groups. Only 6.8 per cent of users are enrolled in groups with a ratio of 3.1 members per group, and just 38 per cent of these groups have posted any document since 2014. In addition, 31 per cent of the documents in the system are included in groups. This low participation in groups interacting directly with other users suggests that Mendeley is used more as an information source than as a networking site. The recent survey by Nature has already suggested this may be the case, uncovering the fact that the main use of the site is to 'discover recommended papers' (Van Noorden, 2014). Other surveys have also confirmed that contacting other users is the last reason to use Mendeley (Deakin, 2014; Jeng, He, & Jiang, 2015). These results validate the hard engagement of reference management tools with social networking environments, as we have already commented on at the beginning of this chapter. Thus, the purpose of the users in these platforms is firstly to organize their own libraries and then to take advantage of the information resources available in the platform. However, as a recommended source of information this utility could be questioned as well, because whether not there is a dense and active network of users posting and reading papers, it is hard to see that these recommendations have value. The fact that 60 per cent of papers have none or less than two readers is a serious problem of trust in Mendeley as an article recommendation service.

Finally, in the demographic distribution of this user network, it could be concluded that Mendeley is mainly taken up by research students (57.5 per cent) from the United States (22.5 per cent) and the United Kingdom (9.7 per cent), and where biologists (16 per cent) and biomedicine (12 per cent) researchers predominate. This distribution confirms that the potential users of a reference management tool are young scholars starting their scientific careers who need a powerful instrument to organize their working bibliographies at the same time as they need to be updated on current literature (Jeng et al., 2015). This broad geographical and thematic expansion of the service demonstrates that the platform has been consolidated into the scholarly community as an example of Science 2.0 bibliographic tools.

4.2 ZOTERO

Zotero is a reference management tool whose particular attraction is that its code is open. It was started by Dan Cohen, Josh Greenberg and Dan Stillman of the Center for History and New Media of George Mason University in October 2006. In 2008, Zotero was sued by Thomson Reuters based on the claim that Zotero can convert EndNote's proprietary styles into open citation ones. However, in 2011, Thomson Reuters withdrew the lawsuit. This fact was considered an example of the attempt of the publishing industry to limit open software initiatives and the free sharing of bibliographic information (Nature, 2008).

The platform started as an add-on for Mozilla Firefox, an open-source web browser (Cohen, 2008). With the correct mechanism into that navigator, Zotero could identify and extract any citation (bibliographic references, websites, books, etc.) that were present in a web page and then store it in a personal library (Puckett, 2011). Unlike other reference management tools or bookmarking sites, Zotero allows the capture of any material: images, videos, snapshots, etc. On top of this, it was possible to include and associate other files to those references (i.e. pdfs, images, links), becoming that library in a personal organized repository. Zotero permits notes, comments and tags to be added to references, which increases their findability and improves the content of each record.

In 2006, it also incorporated different export formats, enabling the collection and export of items in BibTex, CSL JSON, RIS, RefWork and other important formats (Ritterbush, 2007). In addition, Zotero accepts records from Thomson ISI, PubMed, Medline and CrossRef. In 2007, Zotero could be integrated with word processors such as Microsoft Word, OpenOffice and WordPress. This made the insertion of citations and the generation of bibliographies easier. In addition, through the Citation Style Language (CSL), it was possible to build and design any citation style. At the last version, in January 2011, Zotero became Zotero Standalone, a desktop suite independent from the web browser, allowing the collection of references on one's own computer.

4.2.1 References in the Cloud

Zotero incorporated Zotero Server in 2009, a mechanism that makes it possible to create a copy of the user's library in the central server of the organization. This allowed access to this library to be synced from several devices and this content to be shared with other users. In this form, Zotero created its social networking functionalities, specifically groups and profiles, with dissimilar developments.

4.2.1.1 Profiles, Just a Calling Card

Profiles in Zotero only contain basic information to identify each user, with data on affiliation, location, followers/followings and disciplines. It also includes links to access users' libraries and make contact possible between them through internal messages. However, the access to these personal libraries is optional and only a small number of users keep their libraries open source (4 per cent). This makes it impossible to know how many documents are posted in the system. In total, it is estimated that Zotero has no more than 130,000 registered users in May 2015, a figure quite low in relation to other academic sites. This estimation was obtained by extracting the list of profiles from the main page in an iterative process until only duplicated profiles may be extracted.

Zotero is one of the sites that is the most harmful to spam profiles. Some social sites are utilised to insert advertisements or links to increase the visibility of certain websites, improving the ranking of those websites fraudulently when they are searched, for example, in Google. In the case of Zotero, 2,787 (2.1 per cent) profiles were identified as fake users, whose sole purpose was to include links to, for example, online pharmacy stores, real-estate advertisings and escort offers. These users do not carry out any action in the system, but simply make use of the high PageRank of the site to promote their businesses. This is a serious problem because it distorts the normal functioning of the network and affects the statistical analysis of this site.

Not all the profiles are assigned to a discipline and then only 88,455 (68 per cent) profiles were classified using Zotero's own scheme. This system is based on the classification of academic disciplines published in Wikipedia (2015) to thematically organize a user's profile. The scheme covers all the academic disciplines and is arranged in five main classes. However, this system has several weaknesses. The first is that there are complaints of constant and arbitrary modifications with the removing and renaming of disciplines and the allocation of new categories which produce serious instability. Another specific problem is that it divides academic disciplines and professions, splitting related categories into separate parts. In addition, some disciplines are misclassified such as Archeology and Anthropology which are included in Social Sciences. Perhaps due to this, Zotero only takes the main categories without any hierarchical relationship. In any event, this scheme contains five principal classes that make possible the grouping of Zotero's categories. These classes have been re-adapted to make possible further comparison with other social sites.

Figure 4.10 shows the percentage of users by the six principal research areas. As we have been seen before, only 68 per cent of users fill in this information in their profiles. The figure shows that Zotero is unbalanced towards social scientists (33.8 per cent) and humanists (27.6 per cent), whereas physicians (6.1 per cent) and natural scientists (i.e. chemists, biologists) (11.4 per cent) present percentages that are way below their usual representation in other social sites and databases. Therefore, it can be assumed that this population is not thematically homogeneous, being biased towards Human and Social Sciences content.

According to the distribution of profiles by organization, Zotero describes a similar pattern to that observed with BibSonomy (see Table 4.8). The university with most profiles is the *George Mason University* (0.9 per cent), the place where this software was created. *Walden University* (0.7 per cent), a small university in Minnesota, comes second in terms of the number of profiles a

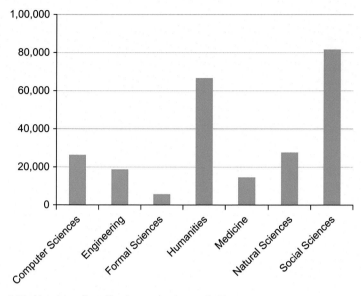

Figure 4.10 Number of profiles by research area in Zotero.

Table 4.8 The ten organizations with the most profiles in Mendeley

Affiliation	Profiles	% profiles
George Mason University	519	0.91
Walden University	407	0.71
Universidad Nacional Autónoma de México	331	0.58
University of Washington	287	0.50
University of California, Los Angeles	236	0.41
Harvard University	236	0.41
University of California, Berkeley	235	0.41
University of Toronto	222	0.39
CNRS	212	0.37
University of Michigan	201	0.35
Total	56,949	100

surprising fact that could be explained by the strong support that this university's library offers to Zotero, publishing an online user guide (Walden University, 2015). As a result of this the students and professors massively use this platform. The remaining universities are common organizations in these distributions, such as the *Universidad Nacional Autónoma de México* (0.58 per cent) and the *University of Washington* (0.5 per cent).

Grouping profiles in terms of countries, Table 4.9 confirms the massive presence of American users – to half of the users come from the

Table 4.9 The ten countries with the most profiles in Zotero

Country	Profiles	% profiles	% penetration
United States	44,067	43.56	2.35
United Kingdom	6,257	6.19	1.66
Canada	3,803	3.76	1.61
France	3,500	3.46	0.94
Australia**	3,224	3.19	2.32
Germany	2,689	2.66	0.53
India*	2,151	2.13	0.74
Spain	1,939	1.92	0.99
Brazil*	1,313	1.30	0.63
Mexico	1,114	1.10	1.61
Total	101,164	100	100

*2010.
**2008.

United States (43.5 per cent), followed far behind by the *United Kingdom* (6.2 per cent) and *Canada* (3.8 per cent). In addition, the *United States* is the country with the highest penetration index (2.35 per cent), which confirms the local nature of this service. *Australia* (2.32 per cent) is the second country according the penetration index, suggesting that this utility has a mean spread across Anglo-Saxon countries. However, it is necessary to take into account that these countries are the most infected by spam users, so these results could be distorted by that malicious practice. With regard to the Country Spreading index, Zotero is the second web space with the highest concentration of population in the first ten countries (69.3 per cent). This confirms the local nature of the site and its weak diffusion into other parts of the world.

Zotero allows users to follow the posting activity of other profiles, promoting the interaction and sharing of references between them. In this way, it is possible to know the number of followers that a profile has and the amount of profiles that are followed. In addition, this number could be considered an indicator of the network's degree of connection and could be a measure of the strength with which the users interact among them. Figure 4.11 shows the distribution of followings and followers by profile. Because the sample is reduced, data were not binned. Both describe a very similar trend, with a slight higher slope for followings ($\gamma = 2.13$) than for followers ($\gamma = 2.16$). However, the proportion of profiles that do not follow anybody is 93 per cent and 89 per cent who do not have any followers. The average of followers is 2.2 while the average of followings is 3.5.

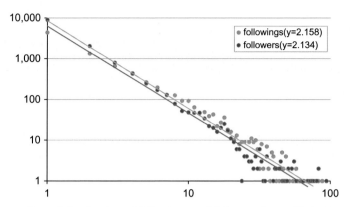

Figure 4.11 Binned distribution of followings and followers by profile in Zotero (log-log plot).

These figures show that the Zotero network is quite sparse and only a small fraction of profiles have connections between them. This unrelated network could be explained because users' libraries are not open in all cases and it is hard to follow a profile that just contains identification data. Another cause, no less important, is the high presence of spammer profiles which show no interest in connecting with other users.

Figure 4.12 shows the evolution of the number of profiles in Zotero since 2009, the moment in which this reference management tool incorporated the creation of profiles by part of their users. These data from 2009 onwards have been obtained from Zotero's main page using the WayBack Machine of Archive.org. Since that date, the number of profiles has been steadily increasing up to the present (CAGR = 76 per cent). The accumulated trend describes a linear growth, with a pause in the increase. Despite the peak in 2011, the incorporation of new users has grown at a very slow rate.

4.2.1.2 Groups, the Only Way of Sharing
In the manner of Mendeley, Zotero allows any user to create groups that share his or her own library with other members. Groups can be private or public. The former are confidential and only visible to members, while the latter are open to any users and allow the exploration of their content. Zotero lists 31,784 public groups in May 2015, of which 64 per cent are open to new members while 35.6 per cent are closed to new admissions.

Table 4.10 presents the ten most important groups in Zotero according to activity. There are 106,597 (82 per cent) users enrolled in these

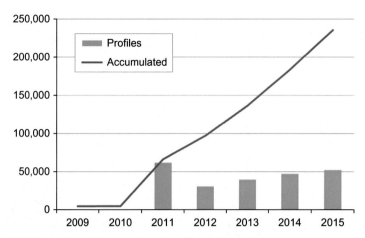

Figure 4.12 Evolution of the number of profiles in Zotero.

Table 4.10 The ten most active groups in Zotero

Name	Members	Items	Activity
First World War Studies Bibliography	60	5,476	91.27
New Orleans Studies UNO	57	4,563	80.05
EEA	60	4,621	77.02
LCENVS	79	5,091	64.44
H–Buddhism Bibliography Project	135	8,298	61.47
GEOgraphie urbaine, régionale et sociale-IGD	63	3,141	49.86
Schulfach Musik Literaturlisten	58	2,885	49.74
DigiPlay	103	3,117	30.26
Géographie-nouveautés BCU Lausanne	109	2,516	23.08
Lidilem	96	2,178	22.69
Total	106,597	2,528,162	23.72
Average	3.35	105.43	40.82

groups, making this the social site in the study with the highest proportion of users registered in groups. However, this figure may not be as high because users can participate in several groups. Despite this, this high proportion would suggest that most of the users only feel attracted to Zotero for its networking possibilities and not so much for its individual functions. However, the users by group rate (3.3) is not that high, which could mean that many of these groups are small. In fact, 41 per cent of these groups have only one member, which could confirm that many individual users are creating groups to share their collections more easily. Observing the number of items posted, these groups in total share around 2.5 million documents, a considerable number in view of the number of users in the system. In line with this result, the average of uploaded references per group (105) also shows that the usage of these groups is high and they contain a substantial amount of documents. This perception is confirmed by the activity ratio (40.8), the second highest value of the sites analysed.

If we look at Table 4.10 in more detail, different groups for distinct purposes may be found. There are groups created for gathering references related to defined research issues such as the First World War (*First World War Studies Bibliography*) or Buddhism (*H-Buddhism Bibliography Project*). These groups arise with the objective of building exhaustive bibliographies that support the research in those fields. Other groups are created as bibliographic instruments for specific institutions in their scholarly activity (i.e. *GEOgraphie urbaine, régionale et sociale-IGD, LCENVS*). It is interesting to notice that half of the most active groups are devoted to Humanities, which confirms the strong presence of researchers from this field of study.

Figure 4.13 shows the increase in the number of new groups since the creation of this tool in 2009. The line shows a constant growth from that moment, but in a paused form. Thus, from 2009 to 2014, groups have grown 60 per cent each year in average. This increase is in relation to the previous results, confirming that this collaborative tool enjoys good health and suggesting that Zotero's users are employing this instrument to interact with other users and the system in general.

Figure 4.14 illustrates another way to look at the positive working of this tool. It shows the number of groups by the year in which users posted their last item. As with the previous figure, the trend maintains a pattern of growth and many of the groups describe recent activity. Thus, 34.6 per cent of the groups posted their last items in the period 2014–15, a similar percentage to Mendeley.

4.2.2 Open Source, Close Content

Zotero emerged into the panoply of reference management systems as a small plug-in designed for an open-source navigator, Mozilla Firefox, and was created to capture bibliographic references across the Web. Since those modest beginnings, this open-source tool has continued to grow and has now become Zotero Standalone, a complete platform that makes possible the storage of bibliographic references and the generation of different outputs (e.g. bibliographies, inserting citations, export/import items, etc.) which can be shared with other members through groups. The main

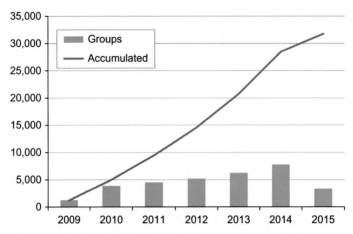

Figure 4.13 Evolution of the number of groups in Zotero.

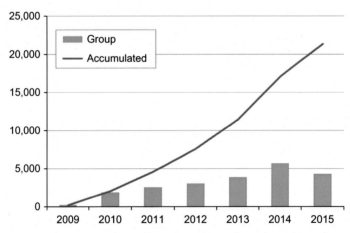

Figure 4.14 Number of groups by year in which the last post was made in Zotero.

attraction of Zotero is its open nature, and the code can be reutilised to implement upgrades and add new functionalities by a developer community. Another strong point is the acceptance of any type of materials, including video, images, audio, etc., which it converts into a multimedia solution to post talks and pictures (Watkins, 2013).

Nevertheless, Zotero lacks of one of the most important elements, not only for a reference management software but for any academic social site. It does not have a public and accessible bibliographic database that permits the browsing of the literature posted into the system. This critical failure means that the sharing of information resources between partners at the individual level is not possible. Unlike Mendeley, CiteULike or other bookmarking sites, Zotero does not publish a common repository from the libraries of their users, which prevents knowledge of what content is being posted to the platform. It is true that each private library may be open to be reused, but the percentage of users that open their collections is anecdotal (4 per cent). This affects the social engagement of the site because many profiles do not have anything to share or offer to the community. Thus the insignificant percentage of followers (11 per cent) and followings (7 per cent) could reflect a situation where paradoxically its greatest problem is the sharing of individual content.

This deeply limits the social networking possibilities of Zotero and leaves groups as the only collaborative tool. It is not surprising then that this platform describes the largest proportion of users registered in a group (82 per cent). It is possible that, faced with an absence of networking tools, users decide to set up groups to be able to share references and other materials. The activity level seems to confirm this assumption as the average of posted papers is one of the highest among academic social sites (105); the activity index (40.8) also presents elevated values and the percentage of update groups (34.6 per cent) is also very high. These indicators suggest that Zotero could be used not as a personal site to manage references, but as an exclusive environment to share references with other members previously defined. For example, partners in a project, colleagues from the same institution or students on the same course could resort to Zotero only for participating in groups.

However, one of the most dangerous scourges that a social website has to contend with today is perhaps the spammer profiles. These users act as a virus, utilizing the platform just to insert advertisements and links that promote their businesses in search engines and avoiding any participative action. Every social site has mechanisms to protect its members from malicious users, but it seems that Zotero does have the proper weapons to mitigate this harm. Although the proportion is not excessive (2.1 per cent), it is indeed significant and it could get worse.

As has already been seen with BibSonomy, Zotero also shows symptoms that its social platform has not taken off from the initial environment where it was born. Hence, Zotero remains a specialized service for social scientists (33.8 per cent) and humanists (27.6 per cent), and is limited to a small local environment in which the highest percentage of users come from its alma mater George Mason University (0.9 per cent) and where Americans form the greatest proportion of users (43.5 per cent) of all the academic social sites analysed. These data show that in the six years this social platform has been running, it has not been able to reach a wider audience both geographically and thematically, which demonstrates that the site has reached a standstill and raises some doubts about its future development.

4.3 COULD A REFERENCE MANAGER BE A SOCIAL SITE?

Reference management tools mark a further step in the evolution of scholarly social sites because they join the ability of organizing a collection of bibliographic references with the possibility of sharing them with other users. Unlike the social bookmarking sites, these new services are based on a hybrid system set up by a personal desktop application that organizes, edits and exports/imports the items included in each library itself, and a web platform that makes possible the sharing of these materials. This converts reference management software into a more advanced product because they are not only a site where references may be stored but software to utilize these items in bibliographies, citations, etc. As with social bookmarking sites, these spaces also aspire to become an important academic source of scientific information. For example, Mendeley contains more than 14 million records in its public catalogue, more than CiteSeerX, which turns it into a bibliographic example for the research community. This brings a great opportunity to compete in the market for academic search engines because these sites have the advantage of supplying usage metrics as well as social tagging, a complementary means for tracking the readership of the articles.

These products have evolved from the local environment of the personal computer to the social space of the web platform. This fact brings a critical challenge, because they have to fit these separate worlds together. Reference management tools, as bookmarking sites, look for the enrichment of their databases in the community through the posting of non-published and multimedia items, as well as making the most of the users' activity when they tag (information management) and explore (usage indicators) their content. This would explain why these products jumped from the desktop to the Web. But it is not clear that this leap was demanded by their users. In other words, there are serious doubts whether their members take advantage of these social environments when they just want to manage their own libraries. Surveys on Mendeley – there are hardly any analyses on Zotero – have let slip that users are not interested in the social networking possibilities of this site (Deakin, 2014; Jeng et al., 2015; Van Noorden, 2014). The quantitative results of this study confirm and expand these findings. Mendeley has proved that there are few individual interactions (median followers = 4), that their users barely share information and documents in their profiles (13.7 per cent) and that very few members set up groups (median = 3.3). In the case of Zotero, the situation is even worse because only 4 per cent of users make their libraries accessible and the interaction rate is insignificant (11 per cent of users with followers). Groups in these platforms describe better health because they act as specialist forums where a reduced number of users (3 in average) compile bibliographies for a class, institution or society. In the case of Zotero, they are the only way to collaborate with other users.

This overview allows us to conclude that, from a social networking point of view, these platforms have not achieved the establishment of a compact and dynamic social community. It is true that the posting of references and the reading of these enriches the system, giving it a significant added value. But these possibilities do not mean that their users increase their collaboration, nor do they take advantage of participating in groups or following other colleagues. The attempt by Mendeley to create a document-sharing service could be a good initiative to energize these communities, and it could become a full academic site by integrating tagging, reference management, information retrieval and document sharing in the same location. Zotero, however, must reorganize its entire approach, creating a real open library of documents posted and giving more prominence to the interaction between users.

REFERENCES

Anderson, K. (2013). A matter of perspective – Elsevier acquires Mendeley . . . or, Mendeley sells itself to Elsevier. *Scholarly Kitchen*. Available from: <http://scholarlykitchen.sspnet. org/2013/04/08/a-matter-of-perspective-elsevier-acquires-mendeley-or-mendeley-sells-itself-to-elsevier/> 10.09.15.

Cohen, D. J. (2008). Creating scholarly tools and resources for the digital ecosystem: Building connections in the Zotero project. *First Monday, 13*(8). Available from: <http://firstmonday.org/article/viewArticle/2233/2017> 10.09.15.

CrunchBase. (2015). *Mendeley*. Available from: < https://www.crunchbase.com/organization /mendeley> 10.09.15.

Deakin, G. (2014). *Mendeley – CSUC Study Results*. CSUC. Available from: <http://wiki. csuc.cat/lib/exe/fetch.php?media=mendeley:mendeley_csuc_report_v6.pdf> 10.09.15.

Gunn, W. (2013). Social signals reflect academic impact: What it means when a scholar adds a paper to Mendeley. *Information Standards Quarterly, 25*(2), 33–39. Available from: <http://www.niso.org/apps/group_public/download.php/11275/IP_Gunn_Mendeley_isqv25no2.pdf> 10.09.15.

Hammerton, J. A., Granitzer, M., Harvey, D., Hristakeva, M., & Jack, K. (2012). On gener-
ating large-scale ground truth datasets for the deduplication of bibliographic records:
Proceedings of the 2nd international conference on web intelligence, mining and semantics. New
York: ACM.

Haunschild, R., Bornmann, L., & Leydesdorff, L. (2015). Networks of reader and country
status: an analysis of Mendeley reader statistics, arXiv preprint arXiv:1504.07482.

Henning, V., & Reichelt, J. (2008). Mendeley – a last.fm for research? *Proceedings of the IEEE
fourth international conference on eScience 2008*. Washigton, DC: IEEE.

Hull, D. (2010). How many unique papers are there in Mendeley? *O'Really?* Available from:
http://duncan.hull.name/2010/09/01/mendeley/ (10 September 2015).

Ioannidis, J. P. A., Boyack, K. W., & Klavans, R. (2014). Estimates of the continuously publishing core in the scientific workforce. *PLoS ONE, 9*(7), e101698.

Jeng, W., He, D., & Jiang, J. (2015). User participation in an academic social networking service: A survey of open group users on Mendeley. *Journal of the Association for Information
Science and Technology, 66*(5), 890–904.

Jeng, W., He, D., Jiang, J., & Zhang, Y. (2012). Groups in Mendeley: Owners' descriptions and
group outcomes. *Proceedings of the American Society for Information Science and Technology,
49*(1), 1–4.

Jordan, K. (2014). Academics' awareness, perceptions and uses of social networking sites:
Analysis of a social networking sites survey dataset. *SSRN*. Available from: http://ssrn.
com/abstract=2507318 (10 September 2015).

Mendeley blog. (2014). Getting connected with other researchers on Mendeley is getting easier! Available from: <http://blog.mendeley.com/academic-features/getting-
connected-with-other-researchers-on-mendeley-is-getting-easier/> 10.09.15.

Mendeley blog. (2015). Mendeley and Elsevier, 2 years on. Available from: <http://blog.
mendeley.com/elsevier/mendeley-and-elsevier-2-years-on/> 10.09.15.

Miller, M. C. (1993). Reference management software: A review of EndNote Plus, Reference
Manager, and Pro-Cite. *MD Computing: Computers in Medical Practice, 11*(3), 161–168.

Mohammadi, E., Thelwall, M., & Kousha, K. (2015a). Can Mendeley bookmarks reflect
readership? A survey of user motivations. *Journal of the Association for Information Science
and Technology*. Available from: http://dx.doi.org/10.1002/asi.23477.

Mohammadi, E., Thelwall, M., Haustein, S., & Larivière, V. (2015b). Who reads research
articles? An altmetrics analysis of Mendeley user categories. *Journal of the Association for
Information Science and Technology, 66*(9), 1832–1846.

Nature, (2008). Beta blockers? *Nature, 455*, 708. Available from: <http://www.nature.com/
nature/journal/v455/n7214/full/455708a.html>.

Norman, F. (2010). From Sci-Mate to Mendeley – a brief history of reference managers.
Trading Knowledge Available from: <http://occamstypewriter.org/trading-knowledge/
2010/06/08/this_is_an_edited_version/> (10 September 2015).

Oh, J. S., & Jeng, W. (2011). Groups in Academic Social Networking Services–An
Exploration of Their Potential as a Platform for Multi-disciplinary Collaboration. In
2011 IEEE Third International Conference on Privacy, Security, Risk and Trust (PASSAT) (pp.
545–548). Washington: IEEE Computer Society.

Ortega, J. L. (2015). Disciplinary differences in the use of academic social networking sites.
Online Information Review, 39(4), 520–536.

Pimasoli (2014) Creating a computer science data set from Mendeley's research catalogue, Pimasoli: Data, Research, Coding. Available from: <https://pimasoli.wordpress.
com/2014/02/18/creating-a-computer-science-data-set-from-mendeleys-research-
catalogue/> 10.09.15.

Puckett, J. (2011). *Zotero: A guide for librarians, researchers, and educators*. Chicago: ACLR.

Ritterbush, J. (2007). Supporting library research with LibX and Zotero: Two open source
Firefox extensions. *Journal of Web Librarianship, 1*(3), 111–122.

Ruiz-Castillo, J., & Costas, R. (2014). The skewness of scientific productivity. *Journal of Informetrics, 8*(4), 917–934.

Van Noorden, R. (2014). Online collaboration: Scientists and the social network. *Nature, 512*(7513), 126–129.

Walden University. (2015). *Getting Started – Zotero Reference Manager – Academic Guides at Center for Student Success.* Available from: <http://academicguides.waldenu.edu/zotero> 10.09.15.

Watkins, A. (2013). Zotero for personal image management. *Art Documentation, 32*(2), 301–313.

Wikipedia. (2015). Outline of academic disciplines. Available from: <http://en.wikipedia.org/wiki/Outline_of_academic_disciplines> 10.09.15.

Zaugg, H., West, R. E., Tateishi, I., & Randall, D. L. (2011). Mendeley: creating communities of scholarly inquiry through research collaboration. *TechTrends, 55*(1), 32–36.

CHAPTER 5

Document Sharing Services

The last step in the evolution of academic social sites, at least until today, are platforms focused on users' own research production, being places where members are able to freely put at the disposal of the network's members the results of their studies. This supposes, in many cases, an alternative method of publishing that makes easier the diffusion of scientific results such as technical reports, presentations, software scripts, etc., that earlier had remained hidden but which now can be discussed and appreciated by the research community. These platforms help many scholars to publish material such as doctoral dissertations, patent applications and data sets that in other times had no place in the academic publishing system. In short, these new sites are proposing a new and alternative way of spreading academic results.

Document sharing services are one step beyond academic social networking because their intention is not just to build scientific information systems through the sharing of references (reference management tools) and the tagging of documents (social bookmarking sites), which leads only to the creation of secondary sources. Furthermore, they are attempting to build an information service centre out of primary sources, the full-text documents uploaded by their members. In this way, social interactions are established, where the viewing, discussion and rating of these materials are the main form of contacting other users and following the updating of profiles and groups.

Technically, these systems permit statistics to be computed on the usage of the platform itself and all the elements that take part in the system. This makes it possible to monitor the performance of authors, documents and institutions and, perhaps most importantly, the definition of indicators that measure the impact of these entities in the scholarly community. One of the biggest attractions for the research community – and therefore one of the reasons for its success – is that users can assess and value the footprint of their research production on the network. Thus users can observe an alternative dimension of academic influence and discover a public environment in which their own performance may be compared with the entire

Social Network Sites for Scientists.
ISBN 978-0-08-100592-7

community. These new metrics are causing a deep change when it comes to interpreting the meaning of research impact.

In this way, document sharing services bring together two key aspects of scholarly communication: on the one hand, motivated by a commitment to the open access movement, a space is provided where the free exchange of scientific results (Science 2.0) can be made transparent, direct and immediate; and on the other hand, there is a reward system based on metrics that measure the online impact of these contributions in the network. Unlike other types of platform, participation in this kind of network is limited to the ability to produce scholarly content. In previous services, users had unlimited capacity to post, bookmark or read any document that they desired to share with their community. However, in a document sharing service users are limited to just uploaded documents created by themselves.

This chapter focuses on two of the most popular and important document sharing sites for scholars. ResearchGate and Academia.edu are the two platforms that are the most attractive and where the most content is made available. The emerging growth of these sites, the novelty of depositing full-text documents and the building of an environment in which the research impact may be tracked are sufficient reasons to analyse in depth the way in which these platforms work and are being used.

5.1 RESEARCHGATE

ResearchGate was launched by Ijad Madisch, Sören Hofmayer and Horst Fickenscher, a group of physicians interested in the scientific collaboration in Science 2.0 environments. They met at Harvard University and then they moved to Berlin where they founded the platform in 2008. As they claim, their principal mission is to put researchers in touch all over the world, making it easy to share documents and information between them as a way to promote scientific collaboration. In order to accomplish this objective, ResearchGate allows users to create a personal profile where they can elaborate a complete curriculum listing their academic outputs. These curricula could be enriched by uploading the full text of their publications in accordance with publishers' permissions. In this way, ResearchGate acts as a personal repository where each user can promote and share their scientific results with the other members.

These profiles are connected with other colleagues in an endless number of ways that make easy the discovery and location of new partners and potential collaborators. Through organizations, topics and co-authors' lists, users can built a network of contacts that allows them to follow the updating of their partners' profiles as well as sharing opinions and criticisms on their research projects. All this is enriched with a battery of metrics at document, author and organization level that enables the interest that these entities provoke in the online community to be followed as well as the assessment of the performance of these objects in the network context. In addition, this platform introduces Questions & Answers, a participative tool where users can resolve the questions and doubts of other members and rate them, providing a good vehicle to increase interaction and promote collaboration among their members.

But perhaps the most interesting instrument is Open Review, a tool introduced in 2014 for the online review of uploaded documents. As a traditional peer review panel, ResearchGate selects from their users a couple of reviewers who argue the drawbacks and advantages of certain papers as well as determine the reproducibility of the study. In ResearchGate, on the other hand, reviewers are not anonymous and each paper can have unlimited reviews and comments. In a way, it is an attempt to create a discussion forum for each paper, where authoritative profiles hold discussion on controversial and revolutionary results.

ResearchGate has also recently introduced its own format for reading the documents uploaded to the platform (ResearchGate, 2015a). This format allows any document to be structured in sections and the lines edited, highlighting parts of the text. Of most interest is that each user can mark and comment on any text as a way to discuss, praise or criticize certain sections and paragraphs.

5.1.1 Metrics, Tracking the User Actions

ResearchGate introduces several statistics that describe the impact of organizations, profiles or publications on the network. These indicators could be divided into three categories: bibliometric indicators, usage and connectivity measurements. The first (RG Score, Impact Points, Citations and Publications) are addressed to measure the scientific impact and production of each profile. Although Citations are measured at the paper level, the rest are only calculated at the profile level. The usage statistics (Views and Dowloads) are also observed at the paper level and measure the utilization that the ResearchGate community makes of the uploaded references and documents in the system. Finally, connectivity indices (Followers and Followings) describe the contact activity between the members. To analyse in depth the characteristics of these indicators and describe their distributions, a sample of 1.1 million profiles were harvested in June 2015 and their RG Scores, Impact Points, Publications, Followings and Followers were extracted. Citations, Views and Downloads were analysed at the document level so another crawl of 1.2 million papers was carried out at the same date.

5.1.1.1 RG Score

Created in 2012, the RG Score is the star indicator of the site because it is fed by the other measures that ResearchGate calculates (ResearchGate, 2012). It takes into account both the contributions that each user makes to the system (publications, requests, etc.) and the perception in the community of his or her contributions (profile views, document downloads, citations, etc.). The RG Score is a weighted index based on Google's PageRank, in which the score of each user can be transferred to other colleagues through these interactions. This means that not all the contacts between users have the same value. For instance, a citation from a researcher with a very high RG Score is more important than the same from several users with a low score. In this way, the RG Score is a measurement that inspires the uploading of contents as well as valuing the use that the ResearchGate community makes of those materials.

ResearchGate only computes the RG Score in profiles that have made any contribution (posting a paper, answering a question or being followed by others). However, recent studies have shown that the research impact of the author's publications is the element that contributes most in the calculation of this indicator (Jordan, 2015; Ortega, 2015a). In fact, it has been observed that, in most of the cases (96 per cent), this metric is calculated only if the authors have Impact Points. For the rest, the RG Score comes from important networking activity (i.e. Followers, Questions & Answers, etc.).

Figure 5.1 shows the distribution of the RG Score of 660,283 (64.6 per cent) profiles in a binned log-log graph to clearly observe its complex trend. The RG Score is measured in a logarithmic scale so the initial phase of the distribution follows a linear fit, then from the RG Score >60 this trend acquires an irregular pattern close to a power law slope. This means that values below 60 (98 per cent) are stable scores influenced by a limited number of factors and suggests that the greater part of the RG Score values comes almost exclusively from the research impact (Impact Points and Citations). The rest could be unpredictable scores subject to multiple factors, where the number of followers/followings, views, downloads and questions acquire most relevancy.

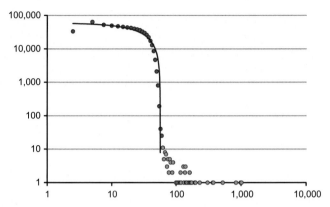

Figure 5.1 Binned distribution of RG Scores in ResearchGate (log-log plot; bin = 2.5).

5.1.1.2 Impact Points

This is another in-house indicator that measures the research impact of the profiles according the journals that publish their works. This index is the result of the aggregation of the Impact Factors (IF) of the multiple journals in which each article was published. For example, a user with a paper published in journal A (IF = 4.5) and other in journal B (IF = 1.5) obtains an aggregate Impact Point of 6. The Impact Factor is a proprietary indicator designed by Garfield (1999) for the Science Citation Index and is now integrated into the Web of Science of Thomson Reuters. This bibliometric index calculates the ratio of citations per articles published during the preceding two years and is used to value the quality of the journals indexed in Web of Science.

However, ResearchGate reveals a technical problem when it calculates this indicator. The IF is a volatile index that is updated each year and published in the Journal Citation Report. When a reference is added to the system, ResearchGate assigns the current IF of the journal independently when the paper was published. Thus a paper published, for example, in 2010 but not registered until now in the platform acquires the current IF when it should have the IF of 2010. Although this failure is not very serious, it has to be taken into account when this indicator is used for research evaluation. Nevertheless, this metric does present some conceptual problems. The first limitation is that IF is an indicator that measures the impact of journals but not of individual articles, because the impact of an article could be very different to the quality of a journal (Hicks, Wouters, Waltman, de Rijcke, & Rafols, 2015). This problem is even more important when only a fraction of journals have an IF and it excludes non-journal contributions such as books, patents and technical reports. This metric could overemphasize the real impact of an author's publications and attribute an unreal appreciation of his or her career.

5.1.1.3 Citations

ResearchGate has the ability to extract citations from papers uploaded to the service. This platform is the first and only academic social network that has introduced this indicator to assess both papers and profiles. However, only 24 per cent of the references have a full-text copy attached, so the number of citations is lower than other citation indexes (Ortega, 2015b), which suggests that this service only gathers a small proportion of the overall impact of these papers. Nevertheless, the high increase in full-text papers is predictive of the growing importance of ResearchGate as a site for the evaluation of bibliometric research.

Figure 5.2 plots the distribution of citations per document in a binned logarithmic scale. This distribution follows a power law with a pronounced trend ($\gamma = 2.65$). This means that the distribution of citations is highly skewed, with 63 per cent of the articles found to receive less than 10 citations and 35 per cent not receiving any. This proportion of uncited documents is higher than in other studies (~20–30 per cent) (Garfield, 1998; Glänzel & Moed, 2002; Van Raan, 2005). However, it could mainly be due to the fact that ResearchGate takes the citations from full-text papers and these make up only 24 per cent of the total database.

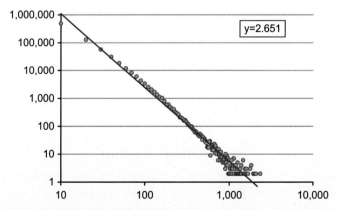

Figure 5.2 Binned distribution of citations by document in ResearchGate (log-log plot; bin = 10).

5.1.1.4 Publications

This measurement counts the number of items that each user has in his or her profile. This is an indicator of productivity and is related to the ability of a researcher to create scientific content. As a result of this, the number of profiles with some documents (68.6 per cent) is rather low which could point, on the one hand, to the existence of non-productive profiles (i.e. professionals, pre-graduate students) or, on the other hand, to inactive profiles without any contribution to the network.

Figure 5.3 presents the distribution of documents per user. As with citations, it follows a power law trend ($\gamma = 2.88$) in which a reduced number of members produce a large amount of papers, while the majority of the users just deliver a few. In fact, 41 per cent of the profiles publish less than ten articles, while 5 per cent of users put more than 150 documents into the platform. On average, 35.5 document references are added by members.

5.1.1.5 Views

ResearchGate also counts the number of times access is made to a document by other members. This is a usage indicator that attempts to measure the early interest that a document provokes in the system, independent of whether there is a full-text copy of it. From the sample, only 17,952 (1.6 per cent) papers have not received any visit, with an average of 85.1 views per document.

Figure 5.4 graphs the distribution of views in a log-log plot. The observed trend follows two different patterns. The initial stage describes a

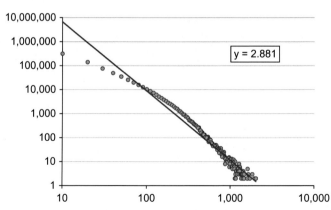

Figure 5.3 Binned distribution of documents by profile in ResearchGate (log-log plot; bin = 10).

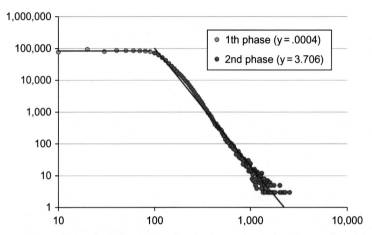

Figure 5.4 Binned distribution of views by document in ResearchGate (log-log plot; bin = 10).

very paused power law distribution ($\gamma = 0.0004$), or a Zipf's distribution. This means that the less visited papers (<90 views) are randomly distributed, showing that a page visited 90 times is as frequent as a page visited only once. This type of distribution emerges when we are studying usage phenomena (visits to web pages, use of words in a text, etc.) (Nielsen, 1997), in which the principle of least effort determines a small number of elections (Zipf, 1949). The second part of the distribution acquires a classical power law with a very pronounced slope ($\gamma = 3.7$), where a small fraction of pages receive an enormous amount of visits. Thus only 3.8 per cent of documents accumulate more than 10,000 views. From a research evaluation point of view and according to the peculiarity of this distribution, we could state that an article needs more than the threshold of 90 views for it to be considered a paper that has achieved some impact in the ResearchGate's community.

5.1.1.6 Downloads

A similar usage indicator is the number of downloads of full-text copies are both deposited in ResearchGate and accessible from an external source such as repositories, open journals, etc. This measure could be more precise than views, because the downloading of an article could implicate a higher appreciation of its content and a later precise utilization. From documents with a full-text copy (48.8 per cent), only 11,126 (2 per cent) have not been downloaded to date.

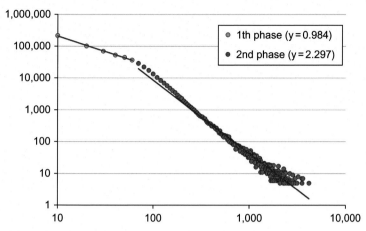

Figure 5.5 Binned distribution of downloads by full-text document in ResearchGate (log-log plot; bin = 10).

The distribution of downloads follows a pattern similar to views as it describes a similar phenomenon: the use by part of the members of the uploaded texts (Figure 5.5). In the case of downloads the initial trend is less paused ($\gamma = 0.98$) than in views, which could mean that the download of a document is less the result of chance and more an intentional act than in the case of visits. In this starting section (<60) there is now more differences in the proportion of downloads, but with fewer orders of magnitude. However, it is in the second phase when the distribution is strongly skewed again ($\gamma = 2.29$) and where the papers with more downloads are concentrated. In specific terms, only 1.6 per cent receive more than 10,000 downloads.

5.1.1.7 Followers/followings

The last metric that ResearchGate counts is the number of followers/followings that a profile has in the system. A follower is a user that stays abreast of the updates of other profiles, tracking new papers and looking out for recent questions and actions. In this context, the number of followers in a profile could be considered an indicator of academic prestige – if users are watching out for the activities of other members it is because they are considered interesting and worth following. On the contrary, the number of followings in a profile points to the networking ability of that user and his or her commitment to taking advantage of documents that other members provide.

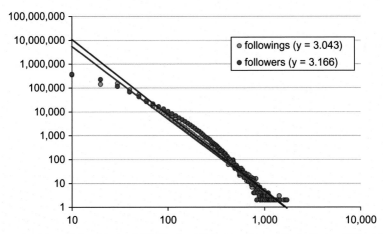

Figure 5.6 Binned distribution of followings/followers by profile in ResearchGate (log-log plot; bin = 10).

Although the before measurements can be aggregated at the profile level, followings and followers are the only measurements of the direct performance of a user in the network. While it is true that articles also have followers who track their research impact across time, the use of this functionality is anecdotal and only 7,907 (0.6 per cent) documents from the sample have some followers.

Figure 5.6 plots the log–log distribution of followers and followings by member. From the sample, 79 per cent users follow some profiles with an average of 25 followings per user, while 87 per cent of users have some followers with 28.5 followers on average. This slightly higher presence of followers by users had already been observed in other academic social sites (Ortega, 2015b), and suggests that while following a profile is a random process motivated by access to information and knowledge, being followed could produce a preferential attachment process, less accidental and more skewed. This would explain why the trend of followers ($\gamma = 3.16$) is more pronounced than the trend of followings ($\gamma = 3.04$), because the distribution of followings is more equitable and limited, while the proportion of followers arises from a few members.

5.1.2 Organizations, Beyond the Personal Profiles

ResearchGate allows users to select their research place from a normalised and closed list, although it is also possible to manually add a new institution. This platform aims, in this way, to organize and group members by their corresponding institution, with the aim of presenting the academic activity at the organization level. This allows it to provide and compare the social networking performance of universities and research organizations.

These institutions are ranked by RG Score and Impact Points. In this ranking, a total list of 44,183 universities as well as research centres, companies, foundations and scientific associations were presented in June 2015. This list only includes institutions with an RG Score, which means this list may not be entirely complete. Each institution has a home page that summarizes their principal statistics, such as number of papers, members, RG Score and Impact Points (Thelwall & Kousha, 2015). However, not all the institutions in the ranking have their own page. From the initial list, only 20,762 (47 per cent) have an own page, and according to the remaining institutions, ResearchGate claims that it is 'crunching' the data of those organizations. This means that there is a post-process of normalization and cleaning of research institutions to avoid duplicates and group organizations under principal entities. Even so, by exploring this list it is possible to observe that there are research institutes disassociated from their headquarters (i.e. Max-Planck-Institut für die Physik des Lichts).

In spite of this effort, ResearchGate suffers the same problems as academic information systems that try to group their content by normalised organizations (i.e. Microsoft Academic Search) (Ortega, 2014). In the case of ResearchGate, each member can only belong to one organization, which produces problems with authors with several affiliations or members that have been moved across different organizations. In that case, ResearchGate groups the production of those authors under the current organization, independently of whether the user's documents were published under another affiliation. This, from a research evaluation view, generates the wrong perception of the societal performance of an organization, assigning it a distorted production and impact.

Another limitation is that not all the members are linked to an organization. Taking a random sample of 1,000 profiles, only 16 per cent were ascribed to an institution. These could be independent researchers or members that do not want to link their profiles to an organization. In any case, this percentage suggests that a significant percentage of members do not contribute to their organizations, meaning that the perception on these organizations is not completely exact.

Table 5.1 shows the ten most relevant organizations by RG Score. A total of 4.2 million (61 per cent) users are linked to the first 20,762 organizations. The rest could be members linked to small institutions

Table 5.1 The ten most important organizations by RG Score in ResearchGate

Organization	RG Score	Users	Impact points	Publications
Chinese Academy of Sciences	226,567	22,077	266,176	94,529
University of São Paulo	153,947	20,072	122,645	54,809
University of Michigan	118,584	9,895	347,274	91,277
Russian Academy of Sciences	115,893	8,369	127,502	73,670
French National Centre for Scientific Research	110,287	5,417	342,700	95,225
Italian National Research Council	108,470	5,620	56,486	17,919
University of Washington Seattle	104,149	8,502	481,766	106,316
Stanford University	101,449	7,735	406,949	88,125
University of Toronto	101,396	10,498	371,332	96,946
University College London	96,211	9,864	226,205	51,311
Total	34,141,168	4,273,172	66,971,882	21,220,277

without a homepage or authors that have decided not to connect with an academic institution. Both RG Score and Impact Points are calculated by aggregation of profiles, so it is natural that large organizations in terms of the number of workers have high positions in the ranking. Among the highest of these are the *Chinese Academy of Sciences* (226,567), the *University of São Paulo* (153,947) and the *University of Michigan* (118,584). However, in terms of the number of publications the rankings change considerably, with the *University of California, Los Angeles* (112,015) as the organization with most papers, followed by the *University of Tokyo* (107,277) and the *University of Washington, Seattle* (106,316).

Grouping these institutions by country, Table 5.2 presents the ten most important countries by RG Score. The *United States* (8.8 million) stands out in first place with an RG Score four times that of the second, the *United Kingdom* (2.2 million). This proportion remains the same according to members, with 22.8 per cent for the *United States*, 7.6 for the *United Kingdom* and 5.9 per cent for *India*. In terms of publications, these differences are even larger with 34 per cent for the *United States*, 6.8 per cent for *Japan* and 6.6 per cent for the *United Kingdom*. With regard to the penetration index, it is interesting to note that it is western countries which show most penetration, such as the *United Kingdom* (2.04), *Australia* (2.02) and *Italy* (1.9). One particular point to note is that *Germany*, a country in

Table 5.2 The ten most important countries by RG Score in ResearchGate

Country	RG Score	Impact points	Members	Members %	Publications	Publications %	Penetration
United States	8,865,227	28,448,927	973,699	22.8	7,224,165	34.0	1.23
United Kingdom	2,237,480	5,215,306	325,231	7.6	1,402,364	6.6	2.04
Germany	1,944,623	3,868,543	195,870	4.6	1,204,637	5.7	0.91
Italy	1,749,779	2,359,904	127,314	3.0	776,387	3.7	1.90
France	1,594,640	2,393,883	129,310	3.0	710,767	3.3	0.82
China	1,526,726	1,991,507	189,722	4.4	956,349	4.5	0.23
Spain	1,268,380	1,580,814	116,152	2.7	539,951	2.5	1.41
Japan	1,239,454	3,934,946	80,862	1.9	1,438,779	6.8	0.19
Canada	1,151,952	2,710,732	130,766	3.1	833,301	3.9	1.31
Australia*	1,008,106	1,584,452	118,292	2.8	500,787	2.4	2.02
Total	34,141,169	66,971,883	4,273,172	100	21,220,277	100	100

*2010.

which the service is located, presents a penetration below one, which indicates that the service is not as popular as might be expected. The Country Spreading percentage shows that these ten countries contain only 56 per cent of the total population of ResearchGate, which tells us that the service has expanded across the world and its users come from a more varied number of countries.

5.1.3 Publications, Self-archiving Driving Force

ResearchGate is fed from the bibliographic references included in institutional and thematic repositories around the world. Through the Open Archive Initiative (OAI), a range of standards and protocols that assure the interoperability of digital libraries and the sharing of bibliographic data, ResearchGate extracts and harvests the bibliographic metadata of the documents deposited in such archives. Specifically, the OAI Protocol for Metadata Harvesting (OAI-PMH) functionality is used to gather this information. These documents are then suggested to existing profiles, perhaps because one of the authors has a similar name to that in the profile. Alternatively, these references may simply be deposited in the ResearchGate database waiting to be required by a future profile (Murray, 2014).

In addition to collecting bibliographic metadata, since 2009 ResearchGate has incorporated a self-archiving service that permits researchers to share the full-text of their publications directly on the platform. To avoid copyright infringements, the platform links each journal with the Sherpa/RoMEO database of publishers' policies on copyright and self-archiving.

Overall, ResearchGate has gathered approximately 80 million documents, of which 19 million (24 per cent) are full-texts (ResearchGate, 2015b). A sample of 1.2 million documents was retrieved from the directory of publications (http://www.researchgate.net/directory/publications). This directory contained around 13 million documents as of June 2015 and provides a selection of the most recent documents to be added to the system. Only papers that start with the letter 'a' were selected for the sample. This list of papers was taken from the directory because it is the easiest way to collect a large amount of papers indexed in ResearchGate, although the procedure could introduce some bias as this list only references the most recent papers in the database.

Thus, for example, Figure 5.7 describes the evolution of the posting of full-text documents in ResearchGate. Although ResearchGate has acted as a self-archiving service since 2009, the sample only includes documents

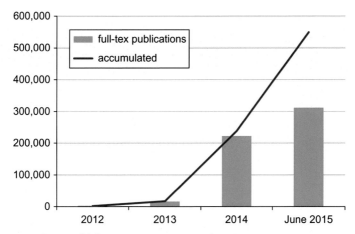

Figure 5.7 Evolution of full-text papers in ResearchGate.

uploaded from 2012. Therefore, according to this sample, 48.8 per cent of documents have a full-text version, just double the proportion reported in the official fact sheet (ResearchGate, 2015b). This means that the more recent a document is, the higher is the probability of finding a full-text copy of it. Hence, during this period (2012–15), more than half the full-text papers (56 per cent) were only posted during the first six months of 2015, the growth rate in this period being CAGR = 320 per cent. These results demonstrate that the archiving of full-text documents is increasing exponentially and it is possible that this trend will continue to broaden its percentages.

Considering in detail the relationship between bibliographic references and full-text documents, Table 5.3 shows this comparison according to the type of document. Overall, *Article* is the most important category and constitutes 84 per cent of the entries in ResearchGate, followed by *Conference Paper* (12.9 per cent). The rest of the categories are testimonials with very small percentages. However, when the proportion of references with/without full-text copy is considered, *Article* (43.8 per cent) and *Conference Paper* (46.3 per cent) are the document types that are less freely accessible, while the majority of *Technical Report* (93 per cent) and *Patent* (91.1 per cent) are full-text copies. This could be the result of copyright restrictions imposed by the scientific publishers that would limit the uploading of papers on the part of users. In spite of this, *Article* (81.6 per cent) and *Conference Paper* (13.3 per cent) are the document types with the most full-text documents. Among the document types, it is interesting

Table 5.3 Distribution of publications and full-text documents by document type in ResearchGate

Total	Articles	%	Full-text	Articles	%	Full-text %
Article	1,022,040	84.0	Article	448,115	81.6	43.8
Conference Paper	157,329	12.9	Conference Paper	72,850	13.3	46.3
Chapter	14,346	1.2	Chapter	9,834	1.8	68.5
Dataset	14,173	1.2	Dataset	11,093	2.0	78.3
Book	2,987	0.2	Book	2,341	0.4	78.4
Thesis	2,440	0.2	Thesis	2,036	0.4	83.4
Technical Report	1,866	0.2	Technical Report	1,735	0.3	93.0
Research	982	0.1	Research	735	0.1	74.8
Patent	548	0.0	Patent	499	0.1	91.1
Total	1,216,711	100		549,238	100	45.1

to comment on the *Research* category. This corresponds to unpublished papers to which ResearchGate gives a DOI generated by its own site. In this respect, ResearchGate is acting as a publisher as well, so that draft and unpublished materials can be read by the scientific community as well as their impact tracked through the ResearchGate indicators.

ResearchGate does not classify its publications by any subject-matter classification system. Therefore the journal titles in the sample were matched with the classified list of journals held by Scopus, one of the largest and most important citation indexes, obtaining 604,502 (58.7 per cent) articles classified according the Scopus subject areas.

The thematic distribution of ResearchGate's publications database will be explored in this way. Figure 5.8 shows the distribution of publications and full-text documents by the five main subject areas, along with the percentage of full text files in each area. In general, 43 per cent of references have a full-text copy attached. *Physical Sciences* (38.6 per cent) and *Life Sciences* (26.1 per cent) are the areas to which most publications contribute, while *Social Sciences and Humanities* (9.2 per cent) and *General* (0.7 per cent) are the disciplines that have the fewest documents in this academic site. According to full text papers, the proportion is similar to previous results, with 35.8 per cent of documents for *Physical Sciences* and 29.8 per cent for *Life Sciences*. However, the full-text rate in each discipline shows that *Life Sciences* (49.6 per cent) and *Health Sciences* (43.4 per cent) researchers upload more full-text papers than authors from *Social Sciences and Humanities* (38.3 per cent) and *Physical Sciences* (40.2 per cent). These results inform us that the content of ResearchGate has

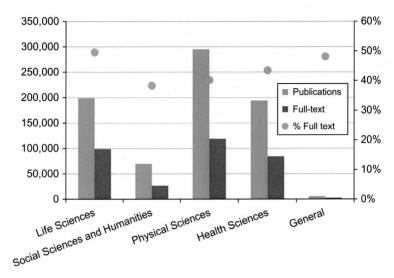

Figure 5.8 Number of publications and full-text documents by research area in ResearchGate.

a clear natural and experimental sciences orientation, while the humanities and social scientists contribute with a smaller output.

Looking at the thematic classification in further detail, Table 5.4 shows the number of documents by subject classes. *Medicine* (17.4 per cent; 17.8 per cent) and *Biochemistry, Genetics and Molecular Biology* (10.4 per cent; 11.9 per cent) are the classes that contain most papers and full texts respectively, while *Arts and Humanities* (0.8 per cent; 0.4 per cent) is the class with fewest documents and full texts. According to the proportion of full-text items, *Agricultural and Biological Sciences* (57.2 per cent) and *Earth and Planetary Sciences* (53.4 per cent) are the subject classes with the most full-text documents; on the other hand, *Arts and Humanities* has only 21.2 per cent of full-text documents. These figures confirm the previous results and highlight the fact that ResearchGate contains more biomedical content than other disciplines, mainly subject classes related to the Social Sciences and Humanities.

5.1.4 Profiles, a Balanced Scientific Community

One of the most important elements in this platform is the profiles of the scientists through which members can interact and share resources with other members. ResearchGate only admits institutional email accounts to create a profile; in this way it restricts access only to academic staff or users

Table 5.4 Distribution of publications and full-text documents by subject class in ResearchGate

Research Area	Sub-categories	Total	%	Full text	%	Full text rate %
Health Sci.	Medicine	179,849	17.4	78,765	17.8	43.8
	Nursing	10,073	1.0	3,920	0.9	38.9
	Pharmacology, Toxicology and Pharmaceutics	26,176	2.5	11,072	0.5	42.3
	Veterinary	5,059	0.5	2,241	0.5	44.3
	Dentistry	4,023	0.4	1,403	0.3	34.9
	Health Professions	7,508	0.7	3,355	0.8	44.7
Life Sci.	Agricultural and Biological Sciences	66,200	6.4	37,889	8.6	57.2
	Biochemistry, Genetics and Molecular Biology	107,690	10.4	52,626	11.9	48.9
	Environmental Science	35,070	3.4	18,311	4.1	52.2
	Immunology and Microbiology	27,329	2.6	13,774	3.1	50.4
	Neuroscience	22,101	2.1	10,597	2.4	47.9
Physical Sci.	Chemical Engineering	25,322	2.4	8,511	1.9	33.6
	Chemistry	61,739	6.0	20,697	4.7	33.5
	Computer Science	56,220	5.4	23,713	5.4	42.2
	Earth and Planetary Sciences	28,996	2.8	15,495	3.5	53.4
	Energy	12,225	1.2	4,137	0.9	33.8
	Engineering	94,742	9.1	33,782	7.6	35.7
	Materials Science	48,452	4.7	17,157	3.9	35.4
	Mathematics	56,026	5.4	23,308	5.3	41.6
	Physics and Astronomy	71,334	6.9	28,407	6.4	39.8

(Continued)

Table 5.4 (Continued)

Research Area	Sub-categories	Total	%	Full text	%	Full text rate %
Social Sci. and Humanities	Arts and Humanities	8,739	0.8	1,854	0.4	21.2
	Business, Management and Accounting	10,706	1.0	4,327	1.0	40.4
	Decision Sciences	9,164	0.9	3,534	0.8	38.6
	Economics, Econometrics and Finance	8,231	0.8	3,506	0.8	42.6
	Psychology	17,707	1.7	8,659	2.0	48.9
	Social Sciences	35,307	3.4	11,998	2.7	34.0
	Total	1,035,988	100	443,038	100	42.8

linked in some way with a scholarly or scientific institution. Despite each profile having to be created by a user, ResearchGate generates automatic profiles (*researchers*) from the authors of the papers indexed in its database. However, these profiles must be validated to be accepted as a real profile. In this study only approved profiles were analysed. Based on the list of organizations, a crawler was performed in April 2015 to gather a wide and random sample of profiles. In total, 1.1 million profiles were identified and their description data and indicators were extracted.

Since the launch of the service in 2008, the platform has experienced tremendous growth, obtaining in just six years more than 7 million profiles (ResearchGate, 2015c). Figure 5.9 describes the annual incorporation of users and the accumulated trend up to June 2015. These data were obtained from the WayBack Machine of Archive.org and the ResearchGate blog. The graph presents an exponential increase of users, with an important jump of new incorporations in 2015. Thus the site growth has an annual rate of CAGR = 126 per cent which predicts good health and massive interest during the coming years.

Figure 5.10 shows the distribution of profiles according to the scholarly position of their users. From the sample, only 376,266 (33 per cent) profiles contain any information in this field and from this percentage, 187,483 (25 per cent) profiles showed a clear academic status. Thus only one-quarter of the profiles includes information on their positions.

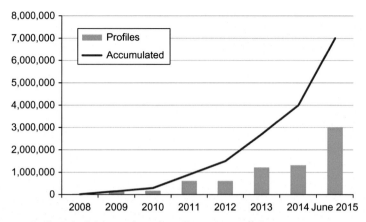

Figure 5.9 Evolution of the number of profiles in ResearchGate.

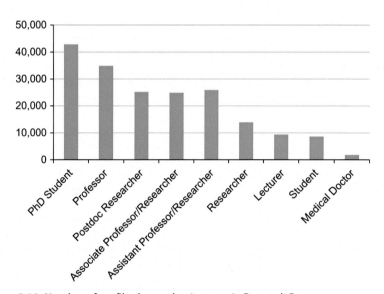

Figure 5.10 Number of profiles by academic status in ResearchGate.

Taking into account only the most frequent categories, *PhD Student* (22.8 per cent) followed by *Professor* (18.6 per cent) and *Postdoc Researcher* (13.4 per cent) are the most common types of academic status in the network. As in other academic sites, young researchers are the group with the most profiles and if *PhD Student*, *Assistant Professor/Researcher* and *Student* are summed, the proportion of starting researchers rises to 41 per cent. A medium age group includes *Postdoc Researcher*, *Associate Professor/Researcher* and *Lecturer* at 31.6 per cent. And finally a veteran

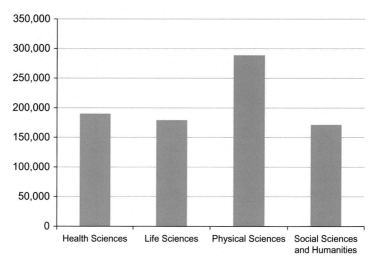

Figure 5.11 Number of profiles by research area in ResearchGate.

group with *Professor*, *Researcher* and *Medical Doctor* constitutes 27 per cent. These percentages are similar to the common distribution of academic statuses, so it is possible to conclude that ResearchGate presents a balanced distribution of profiles according to the age of their users.

ResearchGate permits each member to be grouped by different research disciplines and subdisciplines. In this way, the system is able to orient users towards specific questions and recommend to them new publications in specific areas. Specifically, the system allows the selection of three research disciplines and nine subdisciplines. This also favours the thematic arrangement of the site as well as generating different access points and improving the discovering of profiles. Some disciplinary category is included in 81 per cent of the profiles.

Figure 5.11 shows the distribution of users according to the four main scientific areas. The most populated areas are *Physical Sciences* (34.7 per cent) followed by *Health Sciences* (22.9 per cent) and *Life Sciences* (21.6 per cent). This confirms the high presence of biologists and physicians in ResearchGate, and the less weight held by social scientists and those in the humanities (Elsayed, 2015; Ortega, 2015b).

Looking in more depth, Table 5.5 details the thematic distribution of profiles by discipline. The table shows the elevated presence of researchers from *Medicine* (22.9 per cent), *Biology* (18.6 per cent) and *Engineering* (10.1 per cent), whereas *Religious Studies* (0.1 per cent) and *Entertainment and Arts* (0.3 per cent) present the lowest percentages. This confirms the

Table 5.5 Number of profiles by research discipline in ResearchGate

Discipline	Frequency	Frequency %
Medicine	190,032	22.91
Biology	154,469	18.62
Engineering	84,258	10.16
Chemistry	63,240	7.62
Computer Sciences	44,245	5.33
Psychology	43,303	5.22
Physics	39,323	4.74
Economics	34,325	4.14
Geosciences	26,945	3.25
Agricultural Science	24,912	3.00
Education	24,761	2.98
Mathematics	24,516	2.96
Social Sciences	24,052	2.90
Political Science	8,727	1.05
Anthropology	8,658	1.04
History	5,746	0.69
Linguistics	5,619	0.68
Law	5,591	0.67
Philosophy	3,757	0.45
Design	3,379	0.41
Literature	3,224	0.39
Space Science	2,622	0.32
Entertainment and Arts	2,418	0.29
Religious Studies	1,045	0.13
Other	383	0.05
Total	829,550	100

unbalanced distribution of profiles mentioned above and the preference of this platform for biomedical researchers.

5.1.5 Questions & Answers, a Forum Concealed by Questions

One of the most interesting elements of social interaction is the section Question & Answers (Q&A). This instrument has been through several adaptations since its initial conception in 2009. In the beginning, users were able to join specialist groups where they had a discussion forum to debate their ideas. In 2011, these forums were grouped into Topics and finally in 2012 they were transformed into a questions and answers format (Goodwin, Jeng, & He, 2014), restarting the model introduced by Nature Network in 2007.

This tool permits a technical, methodological or conceptual query to be passed to ResearchGate's scientific community to be solved by their experts. Each query is associated with several research topics and the skills and expertise of members, by which means these queries can be answered by members related to those issues. Queries are treated as threads of a forum, where it is possible to find different answers to a query and in which various members follow how a query is solved by the community. In this way, questions become in turn discussion issues, in which any user can participate by posting his or her response (Li, He, Jeng, Goodwin, & Zhang, 2015).

A sample of 143,349 queries was obtained from a crawler to analyse the behaviour of this collaborative tool and explore the use that the academic community makes of it. Of these questions 94.1 per cent were answered, which is a high response ratio and suggests that the ResearchGate community is very handy for solving this kind of problem. Taking into account this percentage, we can estimate that the total number of queries in the system is no more than approximately 220,000 because, according to ResearchGate itself, 200,000 queries were responded to up to June 2015. In spite of this efficacy in solving questions, the number of users that launch a query is 77,265 (1.1 per cent), that is only one in one hundred members asks a question in Q&A. In addition, 95.7 per cent of these members do not formulate more than five questions. These data show a similar behaviour to previous academic sites, in which only a small fraction of users participate in networking activities.

If we look at the number of answers to these questions, this sample contains 887,868 replies, a figure very close to the 1 million provided by ResearchGate. This means that approximately one in twelve users responds to a query and, on average, there are 6.2 replies per question with a median of 4 (Alheyasat, 2015). This shows that although it seems that the users are a little resistant to put questions, there is indeed a higher propensity to solve the problems of colleagues. Moreover, the high number of followers (1.1 million) and views (56 million) provide evidence that this tool arouses a great deal of interest among the ResearchGate community since many users can find pertinent responses to questions that concern the entire community.

Analysing the relationship between views, followers and answers, we find that there is a good correlation between answers and followers ($r = 0.69$), but views show poor correlation with answers ($r = 0.45$) and followers ($r = 0.49$). This suggests that the questions most viewed are

Table 5.6 The five most answered and viewed questions in ResearchGate

Question	Views	Question	Answers
How can a patient lower uric acid level in his blood without taking any drugs?	366,686	Is Chalmers' so-called 'hard problem' in consciousness real?	5,353
What is the best TeX editor for LaTeX?	165,350	Can ethics be measured objectively?	1,448
What is the relationship between the COD and BOD values in waste water?	124,545	Does certainty or absolute truth exist?	1,104
What is the difference between SEM and TEM techniques?	124,045	Is there a solid counter-argument against Dingle's old objection to Relativity Theory?	970
I would greatly appreciate it if you kindly give me some feedback on this research data management guide	115,352	Are patterns in human designs a mirror of patterns found in nature or are patterns in human designs somehow different from patterns found in nature?	930
Total	56,085,129		881,411
Average	391.2		6.1

not necessarily the questions that receive most answers or followers, and therefore it is possible that there are different types of question that attract more answers or more views. For example, Table 5.6 lists the five most viewed and answered questions in the sample. Analysing the content of the queries, it is possible to observe differences between both types of queries. Those most viewed are queries that aim to solve an uncertainty or demand a simple and direct answer. These queries create sufficient interest but only require a couple of answers. On the contrary, the most answered questions are actually discussion issues that attract many answers but for a specific audience. In fact, many of these queries are related to theoretical and philosophical issues. This demonstrates that the Q&A section works both as a discussion forum and as a reference system.

Figure 5.12 presents the evolution in the number of questions by date of execution. It can be seen that, despite of the service being active since 2008, the number of questions remained constant until 2012, when the number of queries began to grow exponentially up to today.

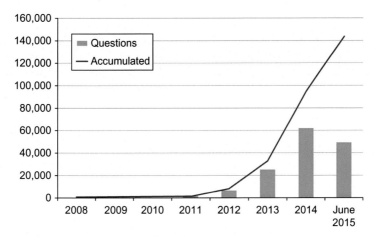

Figure 5.12 Evolution of the number of questions in ResearchGate

This sudden increase coincides with the transformation of the group forums into the questions and answers model, and demonstrates that this change has been fruitful because it has successfully attracted the participation of the community, multiplying their posts and the number of responses (Goodwin et al., 2014).

5.1.6 More than a Social Network

ResearchGate is one of the most interesting platforms in the current panoply of academic social sites, not only facilitating the building of personal profiles and the uploading of full-text documents, but also providing a varied range of metrics that allow members to follow the impact and usage of their academic outputs on the network. Thus ResearchGate connects directly with the altmetric philosophy, puts the relationships between bibliometric, networking and usage measurements in the same context, and enables how they are influenced to be observed. This fact is fundamental for exploring the scholarly meaning of these indicators and what implications they have for research evaluation.

As an information resource, ResearchGate's bibliographic database is fed from a complete list of academic repositories which, thanks to the OAI-PMH functionality, makes it easy to gather an extensive literature. This complements the references that users manually include in their profiles, allowing the collection of more than 80 million references, a significant figure that surpasses the principal citation indexes. However, only

24 per cent of these references have a full-text copy of the document attached, which shows that self-archiving has some limitations. This holding back when it comes to posting full-text copies is sometimes prompted by the disinclination of users themselves and even more so by the restrictions made by publishing houses. In spite of this, the fact that this percentage is getting smaller as more recent items are observed (i.e. 48.8 per cent for papers published after 2012) and that the growth rate of full-text papers increases more and more each year (CAGR = 320 per cent) foretells a successful consolidation of ResearchGate as a document depositing service.

ResearchGate could therefore be considered one of the environments analysed that shows better health as the site also presents a generalized growth in profiles. Thus the number of users has grown at a constant rate (CAGR = 126 per cent), reaching a global spread across continents, disciplines and generations. In this sense, ResearchGate has permeated most countries, from the principal academic powers to new emerging and growing countries. Similarly, this platform has brought together scholars from different academic stages with a balanced distribution of profiles by academic position. From a disciplinary point of view, ResearchGate incorporates an important presence of life and health scientists (44 per cent) which fits with the usual predominance of biomedical researchers within the academic community. ResearchGate therefore represents a growing and unbiased space where a representative set of scholars converges to share their output and prompt interactions between them.

Another outstanding aspect of ResearchGate is the elevated activity of its social network. The analysis of the usage metrics confirms that one of the preferred actions in the network is to explore the research outputs of other profiles (Al-Shara, 2015). Thus, for instance, 98.4 per cent of the documents have been viewed at least once and 98 per cent of full-text items have been downloaded. According to networking percentages, the number of users followed (87 per cent) and following (79 per cent) also verify that following other members is the best way to explore the site's content as well as to keep up to date with new contributions (Chakraborty, 2012). Other interactive functionalities such as Q&A present a high participation with an important response rate (94 per cent), although only a small number of users formulate any questions (1 per cent). All these figures demonstrate the great health of the platform, which counts with a vitalized community that max out all their capacities to obtain the most recent news on their research interests, using all the networking instruments that ResearchGate offer.

One could say that ResearchGate gathers together all the key elements that make the Science 2.0 concept a reality. As a social network, it builds an environment in which the collaboration and sharing of information allows users' outputs to be boosted while keeping up to date in the recent literature, creating a network of ties that stimulate online collaboration and the development of new projects. On the other hand, self-archiving, albeit with difficulty, is becoming a reality that will convert the Open Access movement into an authentic alternative for scientific communication. However, perhaps it is the battery of indicators that is the definitive successful element of this site, incorporating a reward system that brings value to both the bibliometric impact of members' contributions and at the same time enables the online usage of these contents outside of the traditional channels. Along with the RG format, which facilitates the introduction of peer review processes, ResearchGate brings together every element in the design of a different publishing system, an open, transparent and collaborative system in accordance with Science 2.0.

5.2 ACADEMIA.EDU

Another popular document sharing system is Academia.edu, a platform started in September 2008 in San Francisco by Richard Price from the University of Oxford along with Andrew Watkins (Stanford University), Jarques Pretorius (Art Institute of California – San Francisco) and Ben Lund (University of Cambridge). This heterogeneous group of young computer scientists and humanities scholars created this service out of frustration with the slowness of the journal publication process and the lack of access to relevant publications in their research areas (Price, 2012). In this sense, Academia.edu emerges not only as a platform for sharing materials among scholars, but as a real revolutionary Science 2.0 service that wants to implement a new academic publication system based on immediacy, openness and partnership (Price, 2013). This activist support to open access actions could be behind its dispute with Elsevier (Clarke, 2013), which demanded the withdrawal of more than 2,000 papers infringing the Digital Millennium Copyright Act (DMCA). In spite of this, Academia.edu keeps its commitment to the free diffusion of scholarly content and the belief in online networking as the driving force for a new scholarly communication.

Academia.edu is structured into four main elements: profiles, documents, research interests and organizations. These elements are interconnected and allows the grouping of users (profiles) and their outputs (documents) by organizational (organizations) and thematic (research interests) criteria.

5.2.1 Profiles, the Humanists Network

Profiles is a crucial part of the system because through their profiles scholars may build their homepages and upload their publications. This area contains biographic information on users and a list of uploaded publications along with some statistics that describe the performance of these profiles. In addition, each member has access to a personal Analytics Dashboard which details the activity of his or her profile and their publications (Academia.edu, 2012). To analyse the population of researchers linked to this platform, a crawler was designed and performed to extract a representative sample of profiles. One million profiles were harvested along with their organizations, positions, interests and metrics.

Academia.edu is the academic social site that has most users, with 23 million profiles in July 2015. Archive.org's WayBack Machine is used to obtain the number of users at the end of each year but unfortunately this information is only available from 2010. Figure 5.13 shows the evolution of new memberships in each year and the cumulative trend. Since 2010, there has been a constant increase in the number of profiles, the biggest increases being experienced from 2013. In fact, the amount of profiles has grown fourfold (CAGR = 118 per cent) since that point in time. These results show that Academia.edu enjoys good health and its growth phase is still active. However, this disproportionate amount of profiles – three times

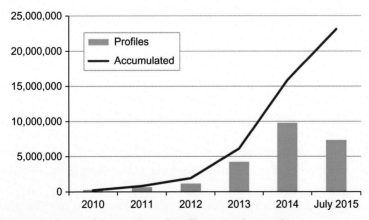

Figure 5.13 Evolution of the number of profiles in Academia.edu.

more than ResearchGate and double the UNESCO statistics (UNESCO, 2015) – suggests that this site is not only populated by scholars, but that it is possible that other types of professionals are using the network to take advantage of the bibliographic resources included in it.

Every profile is able to select his or her work institution from a pre-defined closed list and the department linked to that organization; alternatively he or she may call themselves *independent* researchers if they do not wish to fill in the affiliation information or have simply overlooked doing so. Academia.edu assigns to each URL's profile a sub-domain belonging to his or her institution (i.e. oxford.Academia.edu for members from the University of Oxford). However, these domains are not always correct and Academia.edu can confuse institutions and domains. For example, the web domain of the University Complutense of Madrid is ucm.es, but Academia.edu assigns it emui.eu, the address of the Euro-Mediterranean University Institute (EMUI). In spite of these mistakes, sub-domains describe the institutional presence of profiles in the platform. Out of the 1,010,300 users, only 430,494 (42.6 per cent) are affiliated to an institution; the rest have declared themselves *independent* researchers (57.4 per cent). This high proportion of non-affiliated members could correspond to users with little commitment to the site – they only contribute 31 per cent of documents – or are authors who simply prefer not to provide that information. It is also possible that these users do not belong to the scholarly community, but are professionals and other types of user not linked to the academic world. This fact would explain to some extent the elevated number of profiles.

Table 5.7, according to the institutional distribution of profiles, details the ten institutions with most users and publications. The *University of Oxford* is the organization with most members in the platform (0.6%), followed by the *Universidad Nacional Autónoma de México* (0.55 per cent) and the *Universität Wien* (0.51 per cent). It is interesting to note that there is only one American university (*Harvard University*) in the list, while three British universities take the top positions in the ranking (*University of Oxford*, *University of Cambridge* and *University College London*). It is also of note that among the ten universities with the most users there are two Indonesian universities (*Universitas Gadjah Mada* and *Universitas Indonesia*), which provides important evidence of the penetration of Academia.edu into this South Asian country. Another relevant fact is that there are no research centres or companies in the top organizations, which suggests that this product is of more interest to the scholarly community than to the scientific

Table 5.7 The ten organizations with the most profiles and publications in Academia.edu

Organization	Profiles	Profiles %	Publications	Publications %
University of Oxford	2,610	0.6	27,113	0.7
Universidad Nacional Autónoma de México	2,353	0.5	11,044	0.3
University of Vienna	2,212	0.5	11,787	0.3
University of Cambridge	1,781	0.4	17,350	0.5
University College London	1,564	0.4	18,789	0.5
Universitas Gadjah Mada	1,423	0.3	3,011	0.1
Harvard University	1,407	0.3	10,876	0.3
Universidade de Sao Paulo	1,403	0.3	12,401	0.3
University of Toronto	1,401	0.3	13,529	0.4
University of Indonesia	1,105	0.3	2,664	0.1
Total	430,494	100	3,734,011	100

and professional or that non academic users are grouped under *independent* users. According to the items that organizations contribute to Academia. edu, British universities are those which post most documents, namely the *University of Oxford* (27,113), *University College London* (18,789) and the *University of Cambridge* (17,350). On the other hand, the *Universitas Gadjah Mada* (3,011) of Malaysia and the *University of Indonesia* (2,664) are the organizations with fewest papers. Overall, the geographical distribution of organizations across the five continents provides evidence that this service has achieved international status and attracts users from all parts of the globe.

Grouping each institution by its respective country, Table 5.8 shows the number of profiles and publications by country and the degree of penetration in each. In percentage terms, the *United States* (17.1 per cent) is the country with most profiles, almost twice the number the *United Kingdom* (8.9 per cent) and *Indonesia* (7.2 per cent). As seen with regard to organizations, the elevated presence of the Indonesian members is surprising. This fact is confirmed by Alexa (2015) and Easy Counter (2015) who put this South Asian country in top position with regard to web traffic into Academia.edu. However, the contribution of content is still led by western countries, primarily the *United States* (19.9 per cent) and the *United Kingdom* (10.4 per cent). On the other hand, countries with a strong presence in profiles show low contribution rates such as *Indonesia* (1.8 per cent) and *Malaysia* (1.2 per cent). If the penetration index is considered, there have been no data on Indonesia since 2005 (UNESCO Institute

Table 5.8 Distribution of profiles and publications by country and penetration index in Academia.edu

Country	Profiles	Profiles %	Publications	Publications %	Penetration
United States	73,540	17.1	744,928	19.9	0.92
United Kingdom	38,293	8.9	389,160	10.4	2.39
Indonesia	31,079	7.2	65,439	1.8	
Brazil*	17,043	4.0	116,399	3.1	1.93
India*	15,544	3.6	95,316	2.6	1.26
Italy	12,543	2.9	217,505	5.8	1.85
Malaysia	11,052	2.6	44,220	1.2	3.67
Mexico	10,988	2.6	50,126	1.3	3.74
Australia**	10,884	2.5	129,180	3.5	1.84
Canada	10,419	2.4	117,858	3.2	1.04
Total	430,494	100	3,734,011	100	

*2010.
**2008.

for Statistics, 2015), but nevertheless it may be imagined that this is the country which attracts most users. *Mexico* (3.74) and *Malaysia* (3.67) are the next countries by degree of penetration, followed by the *United Kingdom* (2.39), the country whence comes the creator of the site, Richard Price. These results confirm the wide spread of the service all over the world, mainly into South Asia and Latin America, while European countries describe a low presence, with the exception of Italy and the United Kingdom. This perception is confirmed with the Country Spreading indicator, which shows that Academia.edu (53.7 per cent) is the site with a smaller proportion of users from the ten first countries. It is possible that this massive presence of South Asian countries has only recently occurred, because previous studies make no mention of it (Menendez, de Angeli, & Menestrina, 2012). However, this important presence of developing countries is not accompanied by a similarly high contribution rate as western countries are still the most relevant contributors while developing countries supply only a small fraction of documents.

Academia.edu allows its users to select their academic positions from a predefined list or to add their statuses in an open form. This closed list presents a narrow university viewpoint with categories only applicable to university staff. This produces problems with assignation and many users opt not to put in any information (58 per cent) or insert their position in a free language rather than use Academia.edu's classification (18 per cent).

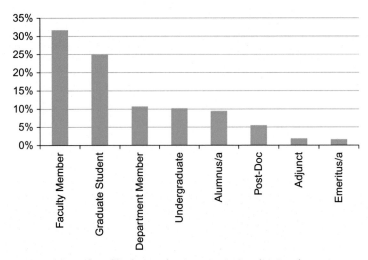

Figure 5.14 Number of profiles by academic status in Academia.edu.

Figure 5.14 shows the distribution of the main categories in Academia. edu's status classification scheme. *Faculty Member* (32 per cent) and *Graduate Student* (25 per cent) are the scholarly categories most frequently found among Academia.edu users (Jordan, 2015; Nández & Borrego, 2013; Thelwall & Kousha, 2014). *Department Member* is the most frequent non-Academia.edu predefined category (11 per cent). In the case of Academia. edu, there is a slightly higher proportion of senior academics (43 per cent) (i.e. *Faculty Member* and *Department Member*) than students (35 per cent) (i.e. *Graduate Student* and *Undergraduate*), which suggests that there is a greater presence of established authors than young researchers. The significant proportion of *Alumnus/a* found (9 per cent) could point to the presence of professionals and other types of users that do not belong to the academic world.

Academia.edu counts the number of times that one profile is visited with the aim of valuing the impact that each author produces in her or his community network. Obviously, this interest is influenced by the number of documents that are included in each profile. Several studies have evidenced the correlation between documents posted and profile views (Ortega, 2015a; Thelwall & Kousha, 2014). In recognition of this, the network presents the most viewed profiles during a certain period of time, classifying them into several percentiles. Table 5.9 shows that the number of items is a strong factor in achieving high rankings, which in turn attracts more profiles and document viewings. Table 5.9 also describes the

Table 5.9 Distribution of average of items, document views and profile views by percentile in Academia.edu

Percentile	Documents	Document views	Profile views
Top 0.1%	39	51,611	2,690
Top 0.5%	27	17,055	1,708
Top 1%	25	9,309	1,431
Top 2%	23	5,746	1,147
Top 3%	23	3,627	975
Top 4%	22	2,626	825
Top 5%	21	2,005	702
Null	9	229	126

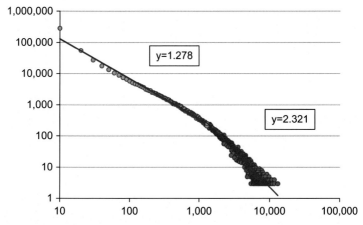

Figure 5.15 Binned distribution of profiles views by user in Academia.edu (log-log plot; bin = 10).

wide differences among users by percentile, thus, for example, a top 0.1 per cent user receives on average 21 times more views than a user in the bottom positions, when this top members contributes only four times more items.

Figure 5.15 graphs the distribution of profile views by user, confirming the observations made with regard to Table 5.9. As with ResearchGate, this distribution starts with a paused power law up to 1,300 views ($\gamma = 1.28$), ending with a pronounced decay from that number of views ($\gamma = 2.32$). This final decay confirms the before results in Table 5.9 and explains how the addition of items greatly multiplies the number of profile views, causing the huge distance between the top users and the common. On the other hand, this also reflects an elevated activity in the site, with an average

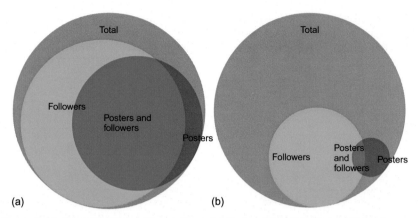

Figure 5.16 Venn diagrams of type of user by their actions: (a) all users; (b) only users with more than five followers and five posts.

of 225 views per profile. This demonstrates that Academia.edu network maintains a highly active exploration of their profiles, being one of their most important actions on the platform. One of the possible reasons for this enthusiasm could be the large numbers of users that are here brought together, which increases hugely the interaction between them.

Analysing the date of the last activity in the network allows us to observe to what extent the actions of Academia.edu's users are recent, thus discovering the percentage of inactive users. This would also indicate the degree of newness in the network and the energy of the users participating in the system.

To extract their recent activities and when they took place, 700,139 profiles were crawled. The results showed that 92.1 per cent of these members carried out some action during 2014–15, so it could be claimed that Academia.edu is in full activity, with a remaining insignificant percentage (7.9 per cent) of possible inactive profiles. However, this activity could be different according to the type of action performed. Figure 5.16 shows a Venn diagram where it is possible to group users with regard to their activities in the network. The results show that there are more users that follow other members (73.2 per cent) than members that post documents to the system (46.3 per cent). Figure 5.16(a) shows a high proportion of users that both follow colleagues and post items (40.1 per cent), which means that most of the people that post documents follow other users as well. However, this is not the same with followers where a significant proportion (45.2 per cent) of these does not post any document.

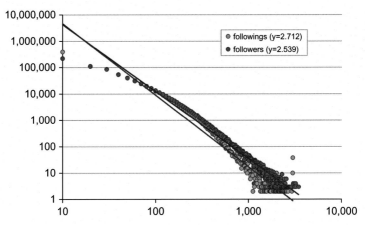

Figure 5.17 Binned distribution of followings/followers by user in Academia.edu (log-log plot; bin = 10).

This suggests that it is possible there are two different types of users: members that mainly follow other profiles and users that principally aim to upload documents. If the sample is restricted to users that follow most (>5 followings) and post most (>5 items), this pattern could more clearly be observed. Figure 5.16(b) describes a pattern of differentiation in which a reduced number of users (1.1 per cent) is very active posting and following. However, the great majority of the most active followers (95 per cent) do not post any documents, while the most important posters (70 per cent) barely follow anyone. This distinct attitude confirms that there is a large proportion of users that only follow the profiles of other authors, and on the other hand there are members only interested in uploading their research output.

Finally, Figure 5.17 shows the distribution of followings and followers by user. As usual, these distributions follow a very pronounced power law trend, with the followings line ($\gamma = 2.7$) a little more skewed than the followers line ($\gamma = 2.5$). Although these differences are not significant, they verify the unbalanced distribution of contacts, in which a reduced proportion of users attracts most of the followers (6.7 per cent of users attract 45 per cent of the followers), while the largest proportion of users only achieve a few followers (65 per cent of users have less than 40 followers). It is the same with followings, which reinforces the fact that there are users focused only on following other members. In any case, the average number of followers (55.8) and followings (37.6) indicate a great deal of activity in this space with averages higher than in other networks.

5.2.2 Papers, an Unstructured Ragbag

Perhaps one of the characteristics that best describes Academia.edu is the possibility of hosting full-text documents in the profile of each user. This site does not establish any limitation on uploading materials, allowing the posting of articles, books, conferences, presentations, talks, etc. In this sense, Academia.edu maintains a full commitment to the Open Access movement and encourages the posting of any academic material on its platform. However, this practice could result in low-quality materials or even spamming practices whether there is no supervision of the content uploaded.

A sample of 688,000 items posted to Academia.edu was extracted from the site using a crawler in June 2015. Due to the assorted range of materials that can be uploaded and that the platform does not feed its system with references and metadata from other sites, Academia.edu does not contain a detailed description of their items. However, not all the documents accessible via Academia.edu are hosted in the platform. From the sample obtained, 404,000 (58.7 per cent) items corresponded to full-text documents, while 29.5 per cent of the records just showed an external link to the document, although not always to a full-text copy. This allows us to estimate that Academia.edu really contains no more than 4 million full-text documents.

Figure 5.18 describes the evolution of the number of documents uploaded to Academia.edu since 2011, the date at which Academia.edu made public the amount of items that had been added to the system. As with Profiles, the Archive.org WayBack Machine was used to obtain this

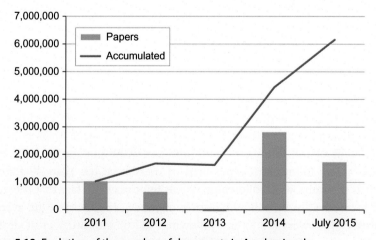

Figure 5.18 Evolution of the number of documents in Academia.edu.

information. The line shows an accumulative growth of items following almost a linear trend. In fact, the annual growth of papers (CAGR = 43 per cent) is lower than that of users (CAGR = 118 per cent). This unhurried pattern could be caused not only by the intrinsic required effort to write a paper, but also by the copyright limitations when a user comes to post it. The annual incorporation of documents includes a gap in 2013, where the number of papers is even lower than 2012. This anomalous data coincide with the conflict between Academia.edu and Elsevier (Clarke, 2013) the latter demanding the withdrawal of 2,000 documents because of copyright infringement. This could have distorted the counting of papers or provoked an in-depth revision of the copyright agreements of the entire database. However, in spite this one-time problem, the system shows good health with 2014 as the year in which most documents were posted than ever and with 2015 heading to improve on that figure.

However, In July 2015, the site contained only 6.1 million documents, a very low number for a population of 23 million users. This means that there is a ratio of 0.2 articles per person, which would indicate that the majority of users do not upload any documents. According to the distribution of items by user in the sample shown in Figure 5.19, only 46 per cent of members post any documents in the site, with 11.7 papers by user. Of these users, 84 per cent have less than 20 documents in their profiles, contributing only 33 per cent of all items. On the other hand, only 3 per

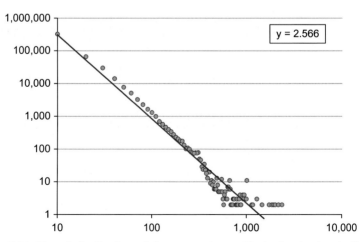

Figure 5.19 Binned distribution of documents by profile in Academia.edu (log-log plot; bin = 10).

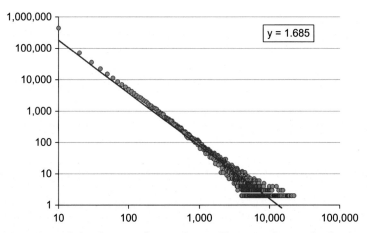

Figure 5.20 Binned distribution of views by profile in Academia.edu (log-log plot; bin = 10).

cent of users post more than 50 items, 38 per cent of all the contents of Academia.edu. This unbalanced distribution would explain the low ratio of documents by user and confirm the strong presence of followers that scarcely post any documents at all.

Figure 5.20 describes the distribution of views by document. In this case, the frequency graph follows a power law with a paused exponent ($\gamma = 1.68$), suggesting the existence of a Zipf's distribution. In this way, differences between a document's views are not so extreme as that observed in citations or documents. Even so, 64 per cent of the papers are viewed less than ten times, while only a small fraction (0.07 per cent) of documents receives more than 10,000 views, 20 per cent of all the views in the sample. On average, each document is viewed 79 times.

5.2.3 Research Interests, Tagging the Content

Academia.edu goes back to a classical element from the social bookmarking sites to organize both users and documents by discipline. Research Interest is a type of tag or label that makes possible the thematic description of the content of each document. There is no limit when it comes to assigning a research interest to a document and, as tags, they are written in natural language, causing the well-known problems of duplicate concepts, multiple variations of the same issue and no hierarchical relationships between them. At the same time, these research interests are also used to group members under disciplinary communities interested in those kinds

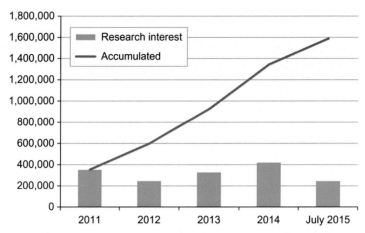

Figure 5.21 Evolution of the number of research interests in Academia.edu.

of documents. To some extent, research interest is a mechanism to put in contact users with documents, which increases the interaction among them and the viewing of documents.

As with Papers and Profiles, Academia.edu counts the number of research interests created in each point in time. Again using the WayBack Machine of Archive.org, Figure 5.21 presents the evolution of the number of research interests since 2011, the first moment in time for this data. In this case, the number of tags per year describes an irregular pattern with ups and downs but a constant incorporation of new research interests each year. In fact, the annual growth of research interests (CAGR = 35 per cent) is the lowest in comparison with documents and users and the accumulated trend shows a linear behaviour. This is due to the reusing of existing research interests, which means that less and less new research interests are created, slowing down the rate of new keywords.

A sample of 510,216 research interests was extracted to quantify the distribution of subject matter of papers and users. Figure 5.22 shows the grouping of the first 500 research interests by four of the main research areas. The percentages provide evidence that Academia.edu is almost entirely occupied by users from *Social Sciences and Humanities* (71 per cent), with *Physical Sciences* researchers (22 per cent) second by far. This massive presence of humanities scholars and social scientists has been pointed out by several studies (Ortega, 2015b; Thelwall & Kousha, 2014) and indicates that Academia.edu may be developing into a specialist social network for those research areas.

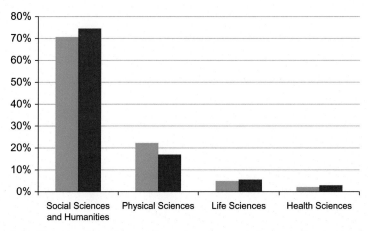

Figure 5.22 Number of profiles and documents by research area in Academia.edu.

Table 5.10 Distribution of profiles and documents by Research Interest in Academia. edu

Research Interest	Users	Users %	Research Interest	Documents	Documents %
Economics	7,053,422	6.53	History	388,193	2.76
Social Sciences	5,949,675	5.51	Social Sciences	336,373	2.39
Education	4,899,775	4.54	Economics	292,751	2.08
Computer Sciences	3,741,377	3.46	Political Science	229,398	1.63
Engineering	3,623,349	3.35	Anthropology	215,466	1.53
History	3,256,982	3.01	Education	199,848	1.42
Political Science	2,729,713	2.53	Engineering	156,903	1.12
Philosophy	2,376,358	2.20	Philosophy	150,019	1.07
Anthropology	2,177,251	2.02	Entertainment and Arts	147,596	1.05
Psychology	1735086	1.61	Computer Sciences	140,918	1.00
Total users	108,036,865	100	Total	14,062,923	100

Table 5.10 presents in more detail the ten most frequent research interests by both number of users and documents. Because there is no limit for users to select research interests, the total number of users assigned to these tags is 108 million, which means that one user selects on average 4.7 research interests. As with Figure 5.22, the distribution shows the

predominant population of humanities scholars and social scientists, and with the exception of *Computer Science* (16.3 per cent), the top research interests are related to the Humanities and Social Sciences. Thus *Economics* (6.5 per cent), *Social Sciences* (5.5 per cent) and *Education* (4.5 per cent) are the research interests with most users. However, Almousa (2011) has warned that humanities scholars include twice the number of interests than chemists, so it is possible that this type of user could be over-represented. According to documents, the presence of Humanities and Social Sciences content is also predominant. Thus *History* (2.7 per cent), *Social Sciences* (2.4 per cent) and *Economics* (2.1 per cent) are the research interests most used to tag the content of the papers in Academia.edu. The proportion of research interests by item is half the size of profiles (2.3), which suggests that users utilise fewer tags to describe their publications than they do themselves. In line with this proportion, it is interesting to point out the different percentage distribution of research interests in users and documents. In the case of users the distribution is more concentrated, with the first ten categories having 35 per cent of the population. On the contrary, the labelling of documents is a little more spread out with percentages under three, suggesting that users tend to tag themselves with generic terms while their documents are described with more specific keywords.

5.2.4 Viewers or Producers Network?

Academia.edu represents a different approach to the sharing of documents, the priority of which above all is the spreading of the results. Although this policy has led to conflict with the major publishing houses, the platform understands that the open and immediate diffusion of academic content is imperative for the progress of science at all levels. This policy has favoured strong implantation in many developing countries, particularly in South East Asia, where scholars have serious problems accessing mainstream scientific literature. It is then possible that Academia.edu is attracting users from these developing countries, moved perhaps by the need to have access to free scientific results. On the other hand, the thematic distribution of profiles has confirmed that Academia.edu is likely to become a specialist network for humanities scholars and social scientists (71 per cent) because they exceed the distribution of profiles and publications. However, there is nothing to suggest that this site was designed solely for the humanities, so this preference only could be explained by the attraction that humanities scholars already registered in the site exert over the new users.

Nevertheless, as a bibliographic repository, Academia.edu presents important technical limitations when it comes to posting documents. The principal limitation is that Academia.edu does not gather the item's metadata in a normalized form, which it makes difficult the indexing of the content in search engines and the proper description of their difficult. This fact greatly limits the visibility of the uploaded documents and could be a serious drawback for the future of the site, because the major attraction of a document sharing site for a scholar is its ability to spread research results. Another limitation is that most of the uploaded documents are not published materials, but in many cases are pre-prints, data sets, reports and drafts that are not peer reviewed and therefore could lack enough quality for scientific research. Although the proportion of these low-quality materials has not been estimated, a manual inspection of the sample suggests that this type of materials has an important presence. Nor does Academia. edu extract citations from the posted documents, making the measurement of the impact of these publications impossible and restricting its power as a research evaluation tool. From this point of view, it is recommended that Academia.edu takes good care of these issues, because these platforms are not just used as social networking sites, but are mainly considered as high-quality information resources for the scholarly community.

In particular, according to the activity of the users in the network, it can be recognized that the members tend to 'specialize' in two types of profiles, those that follow the publications of other users and those that prefer uploading their own outputs. Even though these actions can be done simultaneously, the results suggest that in many cases they are opposed activities which provides evidence of the existence of users with different needs. Thus it may be observed that users who provide few materials may follow many people. These scholars could be considered viewers that use the platform only as an information resource, following a great number of profiles and research interests in order to stay up to date on a variety of disciplines and authors. On the other hand, producers are those users that mainly post their research outputs without making many contacts, waiting to observe the use and impact of their materials in the academic network. This fact would explain, for instance, that a network of 23 million users only produces 6 million of papers, a very low proportion (only 46 per cent of users post any item) that suggests that only a small fraction of users are great producers (3 per cent of users contribute 38 per cent of the content), while the rest are principally registered to read and download these articles. Another relevant fact that sheds light on the disproportionate number of profiles and the duality of roles is that 57.4 per cent of users declare themselves to be *independent*. This could mean they are non-academic members who do not belong to any academic institution and therefore their scientific production is low or non-existent. It is possible, then, that these users are just viewers who take part by following and searching the academic results of the researchers, who acquire the role of producers (Menendez et al., 2012). At the same time, this would explain the skewed distribution of followers and following, pointing to the presence of a reduced number of highly productive researchers that attract a large number of non-academic users that follow these members as the only way to keep up to date.

In general, Academia.edu presents very positive performance indicators, with an exponential increase in new users (CAGR = 118 per cent) and documents (CAGR = 43 per cent) that ensures the continuity of the service and the growth of the full-text repository. This fact should oblige it, even more, to improve its information architecture (i.e. metadata) and metrics (i.e. citations) to be competitive in the long-term. On the other hand, the high activity ratio of this site, with 92 per cent of users posting and following during 2014–15, demonstrates a highly dynamic network with an energized community, although the massive presence of humanities scholars and others from developing countries could threaten to transform this site into a marginal location.

5.3 TOWARDS THE COMPLETE ACADEMIC NETWORKING SITE

Document sharing systems have been shown to be the most successful platforms in the current panoply of scholarly networking sites. The growing rate in both users and content, along with the energized activity of their networks, have shown that this type of service enjoys good health and is catching more and more the attention of the academic community. This promising behaviour predicts a leading presence for these services and suggests that the future of social networking sites is going in the direction of the sharing of documents as a central element in these spaces. This success could be related to the Open Access movement and the search for alternative ways to publish having found in these services a promising instrument for the spreading of academic results. Moreover, as has been seen in the case of Academia.edu, these sites can present a revolutionary vehicle to diffuse content by a part of academic communities under-represented in the main scientific information sources (i.e. humanities scholars) and by researchers with difficulties in accessing the main publishing channels (i.e. scholars from developing countries). In this way, document sharing systems go beyond being a mere social networking place, but are defined as real academic media that are attempting to gather together all the essential elements of scientific communication. It is not surprising that ResearchGate acts as a publisher with its own DOI, incorporates a reward system with usage and impact indicators, and introduces peer-review through Open Review. All these elements assembled on the same site suggests that the ultimate purpose of these new platforms could be to create a new and self-sufficient communication system, independent of the traditional publishing houses, based on free and open access to the academic literature, a *post hoc* peer-review system and an evaluation system supported on both impact and usage.

From the viewpoint of research evaluation and considering their possibilities for an alternative academic publishing system, there are several topics to be discussed that could question their viability. The first is that the quality of the posted materials tends to be low because many are not peer-reviewed. However, in the case of ResearchGate, 81 per cent of the full-texts correspond to journal articles, of which many have been reviewed. On the other hand, Academia.edu does not distinguish journal articles, although it is estimated that there is a large proportion of unpublished material. Another problem could be the incomplete citation count. While it is true that ResearchGate only extracts citations from full-text papers (24 per cent), the exponential increase in new full-text copies (49 per cent paper published from 2012) predicts a greater and greater degree of completeness. In addition, the simultaneous measurement of usage statistics would supply this deficiency, acting as proxy for research impact. Unfortunately, Academia.edu does not extract citations from their papers, which is a serious drawback for research evaluation purposes. Finally, ResearchGate also introduces an online procedure for *post hoc* review of uploaded materials (Open Review), which allows criticism of irrelevant and fraudulent papers. However, Academia.edu also lacks of any type of reviewing or commenting system. Thus whereas ResearchGate is working towards being an alternative to the traditional publishing system, Academia.edu is at present just a platform for uploading papers and tracking their usage.

However, unlike on other academic social sites, users have a natural limitation when they come to contribute content. In a social bookmarking and reference management site, users can post and tag as many items as possible, but the users of document sharing sites can only be active members inasmuch as they are scientific producers. Thus the users uploading the most papers to the system are the authors that most academic documents publish as well. This would explain why the presence of young scholars is not as high as in other social sites, because the scholars who have accumulated the most output are senior researchers. On a different tack, this particular limitation could result in different roles among the users. As was observed in Academia.edu, it is possible that many users are just viewers following and watching the production of other users, while a small number of members, the producers, only utilise the platform to publish their results and track their impact and usage. Somehow, these different roles demonstrate that these online sites can be used for different purposes addressed to satisfy the personal needs of each user. On the one hand, they spread and boost the research activity of the producers, while at the same time acting as an information resource for the majority of the viewers.

As has been said, all this publishing activity is supported by a frenetic social environment, with the best activity rates and the greatest averages of followers and followings. In fact, it is surprising that both sites are preferred more for contacting other colleagues (more than 60 per cent) than for discovering or posting content (below 40 per cent) (Van Noorden, 2014), when the principal objective of these platforms is to become a channel for spreading scientific literature. It is even more astonishing when these sites lack public collaborative tools (with the exception of Questions & Answers of ResearchGate) such as groups or forums that promote partnership among users. On the other hand, following is the only action available to contact other users. However, it is possible that many users follow their partners, not in order to socialize, but as a way to locate valuable information, which would explain the results of Van Noorden (2014). It may be that users search for information following the posts of other relevant colleagues, determining in this way their relevance by authority criteria. This hypothesis is supported by the poor searching functionalities of these sites, with just a simple search window that does not distinguish authors from titles, journals, organizations or keywords, nor do they permit advanced queries to retrieve precise information. Related to this inability to search information could be the absence of groups, the main collaborative tool in other types of academic social sites. In their place, Topics (ResearchGate) and Research Interests (Academia.edu) work as keywords that group profiles and documents, through which it is possible to browse the content hosted in the platform. In this way, this elevated networking activity could really be covering up a serious problem of information searching, instead of being a reflection of collaborative behaviour.

REFERENCES

Academia.edu. (2012). Announcing Academia.edu analytics. Available from: <http://blog.academia.edu/post/29490656413/announcing-academia-edu-analytics> 10.09.15.

Alexa. (2015). Academia.edu site overview. Available from: <http://www.alexa.com/siteinfo/academia.edu> 10.09.15.

Alheyasat, O. (2015). Examination expertise sharing in academic social networks using graphs: The case of ResearchGate. *Contemporary Engineering Sciences, 8*(3), 137–151.

Almousa, O. (2011). Users' classification and usage-pattern identification in academic social networks: *IEEE jordan conference on Applied Electrical Engineering and Computing Technologies AEECT*. New York: IEEE.

Al-Shara, I. (2015). Faculty members' knowledge degree regarding ResearchGate website and their estimations for its effect on the development of scientific research skills of instructors and graduate students at the University of Jordan. *European Scientific Journal, 11*, 13.

Chakraborty, N. (2012). Activities and reasons for using social networking sites by research scholars in NEHU: A study on Facebook and ResearchGate, *PLANNER-2012 Gangtok, Sikkim*. Available from: <http://ir.inflibnet.ac.in/bitstream/1944/1666/1/3.pdf> 10.09.15.

Clarke, M. (2013). *The end of an era for Academia.edu and other academic networks?* Scholarly Kitchen. Available from: <http://scholarlykitchen.sspnet.org/2013/12/11/has-elsevier-signaled-a-new-era-for-academia-edu-and-other-professional-networks/> 10.09.15.

Easy Counter (2015) Academia.edu hits count and more. Available from: <https://www.easycounter.com/report/academia.edu> 10.09.15.

Elsayed, A. M. (2015). The use of academic social networks among Arab researchers: A survey. *Social Science Computer Review* Available from: <http://ssc.sagepub.com/content/early/2015/06/04/0894439315589146.abstract> 10.09.15.

Garfield, E. (1998). I had a dream about uncitedness. *The Scientist, 12*(14), 10.

Garfield, E. (1999). Journal impact factor: A brief review. *Canadian Medical Association Journal, 161*, 979–980.

Glänzel, W., & Moed, H. F. (2002). Journal impact measures in bibliometric research. *Scientometrics, 53*(2), 171–193.

Goodwin, S., Jeng, W., & He, D. (2014). Changing communication on ResearchGate through interface updates. *Proceedings of the American Society for Information Science and Technology, 51*(1), 1–4.

Hicks, D., Wouters, P., Waltman, L., de Rijcke, S., & Rafols, I. (2015). Bibliometrics: The Leiden Manifesto for research metrics. *Nature, 520*, 7548. Available from: <http://www.nature.com/news/bibliometrics-the-leiden-manifesto-for-research-metrics-1.17351> 10.09.15.

Jordan, K. (2015) Exploring the ResearchGate score as an academic metric: Reflections and implications for practice. In *Quantifying and analysing scholarly communication on the web (ASCW'15)*. Available from: <http://ascw.know-center.tugraz.at/wp-content/uploads/2015/06/ASCW15_jordan_response_kraker-lex.pdf> 10.09.15.

Li, L., He, D., Jeng, W., Goodwin, S., & Zhang, C. (2015). Answer quality characteristics and prediction on an academic Q&A site: A case study on ResearchGate. In *Proceedings of the 24th international conference on world wide web companion*. Florence, IT: International World Wide Web Conferences.

Menendez, M., de Angeli, A., & Menestrina, Z. (2012). Exploring the virtual space of academia. In J. Dugdale, C. Masclet, M. A. Grasso, J. -F. Boujut, & P. Hassanaly (Eds.), *From research to practice in the design of cooperative systems: Results and open challenges*. London: Springer.

Murray, M. (2014). Analysis of a scholarly social networking site: The case of the dormant user. *SAIS 2014 Proceedings*. Available from: <http://aisel.aisnet.org/cgi/viewcontent.cgi?article=1023&context=sais2014> 10.09.15.

Nández, G., & Borrego, Á. (2013). Use of social networks for academic purposes: A case study. *Electronic Library*, *31*(6), 781–791.

Nielsen, J. (1997). Zipf curves and website popularity. *Nielsen Norman group*. Available from: <http://www.nngroup.com/articles/zipf-curves-and-website-popularity/> 10.09.15.

Ortega, J. L. (2014). *Academic search engines: A quantitative outlook*. Cambridge: Chandos Publishers. (Elsevier Group).

Ortega, J. L. (2015a). Relationship between altmetric and bibliometric indicators across academic social sites: The case of CSIC's members'. *Journal of Informetrics*, *9*(1), 39–49.

Ortega, J. L. (2015b). Disciplinary differences in the use of academic social networking sites. *Online Information Review*, *39*(4), 520–536.

Price, R. (2012). The future of science. *Academia.edu* Available from: <http://blog.academia.edu/post/22850454488/the-future-of-science> 10.09.15.

Price, R. (2013). After Aaron, reputation metrics startups aim to disrupt the scientific journal. *Academia.edu* Available from: <http://blog.academia.edu/post/42295569220/after-aaron-reputation-metrics-startups-aim-to#sthash.dSb23eYT.dpuf> 10.09.15.

ResearchGate, (2012). ResearchGate introduces the RG Score: A new way to measure scientific reputation. *ResearchGate* Available from: <https://explore.researchgate.net/display/news/2012/08/08/> 10.09.15.

ResearchGate, (2015a). Introducing the RG format. Available from: <https://explore.researchgate.net/display/news/2015/02/12/> 10.09.15.

ResearchGate, (2015b). Fact sheet about ResearchGate. *ResearchGate* Available from: <http://www.researchgate.net/aboutus.AboutUsPress.downloadFile.html> 10.09.15.

ResearchGate, (2015c). Celebrating seven million members and seven years of ResearchGate. *ResearchGate* Available from: <https://explore.researchgate.net/display/news/2015/05/22/> 10.09.15.

Thelwall, M., & Kousha, K. (2014). Academia.edu: Social network or academic network? *Journal of the Association for Information Science and Technology*, *65*(4), 721–731.

Thelwall, M., & Kousha, K. (2015). ResearchGate: Disseminating, communicating, and measuring scholarship? *Journal of the Association for Information Science and Technology*, *66*(5), 876–889.

UNESCO Institute for Statistics (2015). UIS.Stat. Available from: <http://data.uis.unesco.org/> 10.09.15.

Van Noorden, R. (2014). Online collaboration: Scientists and the social network. *Nature*, *512*(7513), 126–129.

Van Raan, A. (2005). Measuring science. In H. F. Moed, W. Glanzel, & U. Schmoch (Eds.), *Handbook of quantitative science and technology research*. New York: Kluwer Academic.

Zipf, G. K. (1949). *Human behavior and the principle of least effort*. Oxford: Addison-Wesley Press.

CHAPTER 6

Comparison

Raw data themselves are not sufficient to get a complete picture of the social activity developed in a networking site, but it is necessary to contextualize these results with other academic social spaces so that we can observe the success or failure of each service in relation to its competitors. In addition, this comparison exercise allows us to observe more clearly how different types of social sites work, pointing out the strengths or weaknesses of each model. Thanks to this quantitative approach, this benchmarking exercise can be more easily conducted because it enables comparison between several indicators and measurements, which illustrate in each case how a model has built up a large inclusive scientific community that contributes genuine value and rich content through its functionalities and services.

6.1 SIZE, SEARCHING THE CRITICAL MASS

A key element in any social site is its size in terms of users and content, because the use and success of their functionalities depends on the number of signed members and their ability to produce contents. Thus, for example, the networking activity or the usage metrics need a consistent critical mass to their results are significant. Thus, Profiles and Publications are the two critical elements that define the size of an academic social site.

6.1.1 Profiles, the Main Asset of a Network

The principal asset of a social networking site is its users because without them there is simply no site. As a result of this, it is not surprising that the owners of social sites are proud of the number of users that they host and celebrate when they reach an important milestone. The number of users registered in a social site is always considered an indicator of size and describes the power of a site to attract and accumulate members. A highly populated network therefore favours networking among partners, the creation of collaborative structures and the provision of new relevant content. To some extent, each social site needs a critical mass to develop these basic

Social Network Sites for Scientists.
ISBN 978-0-08-100592-7
149

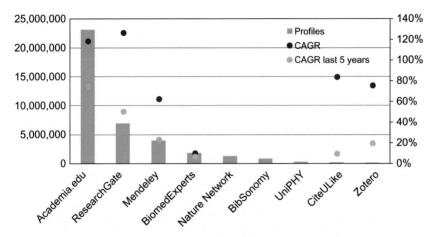

Figure 6.1 Number of profiles and annual growth rate in each social site.

functionalities and begin to attract more potential users, in turn increasing its value. Following Reed's law, the value of a social site increases as more members join that network because the number of possible new groups or connections exponentially increases (Reed, 2001).

Figure 6.1 presents the total number of users registered in each social site in 2015. The site with the greatest number of users is *Academia. edu*, with 23 million scholars, followed far behind by *ResearchGate* with 7 million and *Mendeley* with 4 million. The smallest networks are *Zotero* (130,000), *CiteUlike* (208,000) and *UniPHY* (300,000). In the case of *BiomedExperts* it is necessary to specify that only 471,000 profiles were validated, and in *BibSonomy* only a much a reduced group of users (9,000) remain active. These figures illustrate that, in the panorama of the academic social sites, document sharing systems are consolidating, being the platforms that attract most users, far and above other models such as reference management and social bookmarking sites. Of these, Mendeley is the only non-document sharing platform that may be considered a successful site with 4 million users. The most surprising is that Academia.edu has four times the number of profiles of its nearest competitor. This disproportionate number of users could be due to the fact that many of these profiles may be non-academic *independent* members that are using the site only for exploring full-text documents instead for uploading items.

However, the number of users in a site has to be observed from a temporal point of view in order to properly describe the energy with which these sites are growing and projecting their future positions. The annual growth rate was calculated to measure the growing trend of each site. To calculate this indicator longitudinal data were necessary, so it could not be computed for *Nature Network, BiomedExperts, UniPHY* (no longer available) and *BibSonomy* (without historical data). However, according to this indicator, the sites that present the greatest increase are the two major document sharing sites, *ResearchGate* (128 per cent) and *Academia.edu* (118 per cent), followed far behind again by *CiteULike* (84 per cent) and *Zotero* (76 per cent). This result confirms the emerging behaviour of the document sharing sites and the standstill of the other platforms. It is also remarkable that *Mendeley* (63 per cent) is the site with the lowest growth. For more precise figures an annual growth rate was computed only for the last five years, because the older sites have had more time to accumulate members, whereas the younger ones have not yet developed their potential. Now, *Academia.edu* (74 per cent) presents the highest growth followed by *ResearchGate* (50 per cent), while *Mendeley* (23 per cent) surpasses *Zotero* (20 per cent) and *CiteUlike* (10 per cent), the oldest site. This confirms the rise of *Academia.edu, Researchgate* and *Mendeley* as the three most popular platforms for social networking for scholars and suggests that the other social instruments are losing the interest of the academic community.

6.1.1.1 Disciplinary Distribution

The thematic distribution of profiles is a key factor to observe if the population of a site is balanced or, on the contrary, the network tends to specialize in a specific research area. The specialization could be positive if the site was designed only for the target users, but may be counter-productive for most sites because this reduces the diversity and therefore limits the future growth to see off potential users from different disciplines. Thus if a network does not present a sufficient range of content and there are not enough colleagues in each subject area, then it is possible that those sites will lose attractiveness to upcoming potential users.

Only five academic sites could be classified thematically, the rest corresponding to specialist sites (i.e. *BiomedExperts* specializing in Biomedicine and *UniPHY* in Physics) or platforms that do not arrange their users thematically (*BibSonomy*). Figure 6.2 shows the distribution of profiles according to four main research areas: Life Sciences, Social Sciences and Humanities, Physical Sciences and Health Sciences. This classification scheme is the one employed by Elsevier in many of their products (i.e. ScienceDirect, Scopus) and is used here because it is clear and helps comparison across platforms. *Academia.edu* and *Zotero* show an elevated degree of specialization, with 70 per cent and 61 per cent of profiles belonging to Social Sciences and Humanities respectively. As has been said, the presence

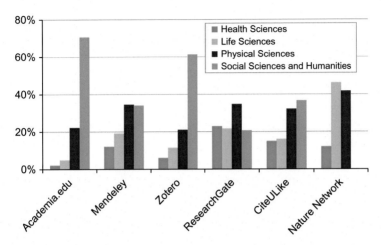

Figure 6.2 Number of profiles by research area in each social site.

of large numbers of humanities scholars and social scientists could pose a risk for the upcoming development agenda, because this fact could limit the attraction of new scholars from other disciplines. On the other hand, *Mendeley*, *ResearchGate* and *CiteULike* present well-balanced distributions with an increased degree of diversification. Even so, it is interesting to note the significant presence of Health Sciences (23 per cent) in *ResearchGate* and the strong presence of life scientists (37 per cent) in *Nature Network* (46 per cent). In this same site, *Business/Investment* (93 per cent), the category of Social Sciences and Humanities, was removed because it could be used as the default class and distorted the results. Due to this, this research area was not graphed for the *Nature Network* case.

6.1.1.2 Country Distribution

The extension of an academic social site across countries could be an indicator of its success in the research community, because as a site grows, it is more likely to attract new users from different places. Thus a service with a large proportion of international users demonstrates that the platform has reached across the globe and become a model for scholarly networking sites. However, a service with a high proportion of local users is evidence that the site has not taken off and has became in a local tool with few prospects.

In this analysis, only *BiomedExperts* and *UniPHY* were excluded because they have disappeared and it was not possible to count the nationality of their users. Table 6.1 presents the percentages of members from their countries in each social site. These are the countries that most users

Table 6.1 Percentage of users by country in each social site and Country Spreading index

Country	ResearchGate	Academia.edu	Mendeley	Zotero	CiteULike	Bibsonomy	Nature Network
United States	22.8	17.1	22.5	43.6	27.2	7.3	32.2
United Kingdom	7.6	8.9	9.7	6.2	10.7	4.0	15.2
Germany	4.6	2.0	6.2	2.7	4.6	41.1	3.7
France	3	2.1	2.7	3.5	4.0	4.6	1.5
Spain	2.7	2.2	4.8	1.9	3.4	2.0	1.2
Canada	3.1	2.4	3.7	3.8	3.3	1.0	2.8
India	5.9	3.6	2.4	2.1	4.8	3.0	11.4
Italy	3	2.9	2.2	0.7	3.3	3.0	1.6
Australia	2.8	2.5	2.2	3.2	3.0	1.0	1.8
CS index	55.9	53.7	63.3	69.3	68.1	73.8	73.6

have in every platform. The results show in general that the United States and the United Kingdom are the countries with the highest presence in these platforms, followed by other western and/or Commonwealth countries. Only in exceptional cases do different countries emerge with better percentages, as is case of *BibSonomy*, where 41 per cent of the users come from Germany. In any event, this important presence of western countries is also due to these countries having large populations of researchers and it is inevitable that they will occupy the top positions.

Next, Figure 6.3 graphs the degree of penetration of each service into a country. This relative index reduces the size effect of large countries with high academic populations. In general, the picture presents a slightly confusing view with a very varied distribution of penetration so it could be said that each social site follows a different pattern. However, with the exception of *BibSonomy*, the United Kingdom stands out as the site with the best penetration across the board, suggesting that researchers from this country show a positive inclination towards these platforms. This could be due to the fact that many of these platforms are located in this country such as *Mendeley*, *CiteULike* and *Nature Network*. The remaining countries present a varied penetration and the aforementioned case of *BibSonomy* should be noted, along with the diffusion of *Nature Network* by Commonwealth countries, in particular India, and the case of *Zotero* with a majority presence of American users.

Another way to measure the spreading of a platform around the world is to measure the concentration degree of their users in many or few countries. Country Spreading (CS) measures how highly geographically concentrated/spread the population is of a social site. High values

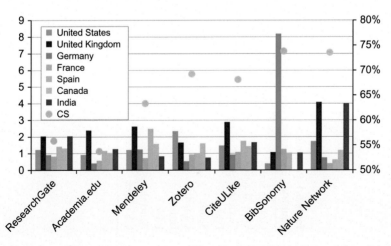

Figure 6.3 Penetration index by country and Country Spreading index in each social site.

of CS therefore describe very local sites that have expanded over just a small number of countries, while low rates of CS correspond to sites that have reached large parts of the world. *Academia.edu* (53.7 per cent) and *ResearchGate* (55.9 per cent) are the services that have spread the most, suggesting that these platforms have expanded the most all over the world. On the other hand, *BibSonomy* (73.8 per cent) and *Nature Network* (73.6 per cent) are highly concentrated in a greatly reduced space. In the case of *BibSonomy* this concentration is around German-speaking countries, while *Nature Network* was mainly instituted in Commonwealth countries. This index could be interpreted as a health indicator because spaces with a wider geographical diffusion are sites with a great development and positive growth as well, as with *ResearchGate* and *Academia.edu*. On the contrary, sites with a small geographical spread have disappeared (*Nature Network*) or remain marginalized to a local environment (*BibSonomy, Zotero*).

6.1.1.3 Academic Statuses

Academic position could be a proxy for the age of the profiles, at least with regard to 'academic' age, because it is common that students would be younger while professors and researchers are likely to be older. It is also true that scholars have different needs and develop different activities according to the academic stage in which they are. As a result of this, the analysis of the academic positions allows us to observe the difference in preferences with regard to the use of one or other type of platform.

Figure 6.4 presents the distribution of users by their academic positions in four academic sites: *Academia.edu, ResearchGate, CiteULike* and

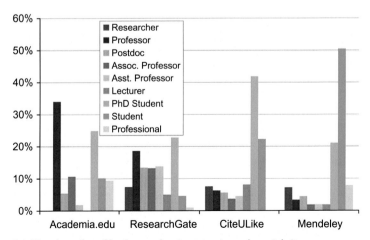

Figure 6.4 Number of profiles by academic status in each social site.

Mendeley. The remaining platforms do not include this information in their profiles. The classification scheme has been developed ad hoc and is expected to cover the great diversity of positions that there are in the academic world. Both document sharing sites, *Academia.edu* and *ResearchGate*, show a varied range of academic positions, with a significant presence of senior posts such as Professor, Researcher and Professional. However, *CiteULike* and *Mendeley*, two sites specializing in reference sharing, present a disproportionate presence of young scholars such as Student and PhD Student. These opposing distributions could be the result of the different solutions that these platforms offer and the type of users interested in those functionalities. Thus, for example, reference managers such as *Mendeley* and bookmarking sites such as *CiteULike* attract many students that need to gather and manage long and exhaustive bibliographies on their research fields to support the start of their scientific career. On the other hand, document sharing sites attract the attention of a wider range of scholars, both younger and older, whose aim is to distribute their academic publications and track their impact in an online environment. In summary, document sharing sites are spaces suitable for any type of scholar, while bookmarking and reference management sites are being used mainly by young students. This, perhaps then, is another cause of the success of document sharing sites over other platforms because they are not limited to a particular age, while other platforms are spaces that principally attract younger scholars.

6.1.2 Publications, Fuelling the Network

If the users are the principal asset, the amount of content that these users contribute to the system is the main wealth of a social site because they represent the results of the activity performed in the network. From an academic point of view, the content of these sites has a very special significance because it transforms these platforms into information resources for searching relevant articles as well as for keeping up to date on the recent literature. Moreover, the social activity of users tagging, reading, viewing and downloading items may be used as an indicator of the quality of these materials, which allows the selection and filtering of documents according to their impact in the online community.

Figure 6.5 shows the distribution of references and documents posted to each academic social site. *Nature Network* is not included because it did not contain publications, nor is *UniPHY* because the number of publications hosted on the site is unknown. *Mendeley* is the site with highest

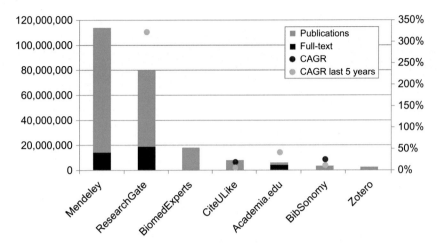

Figure 6.5 Number of items posted and annual growth rate in each social site.

number of references, approximately 114 million being aggregated from all the users' libraries. However, many of these are duplicated and are not publicly accessible from the *Mendeley* website. Thus the figure closest to the *Mendeley* public catalogue is 14.1 million records. In spite of this drastic reduction, this site remains in second place in terms of the number of bibliographic references, while *ResearchGate* is at the top with 80 million references, of which 19 million also have a full-text copy. The remaining services are far behind, with values under 20 million. Hence, *BiomedExperts* contained 18 million documents harvested directly from PubMed. Next, *CiteULike* hosts 8 million citations, while *Academia.edu* contains 6.1 million references and 4 million full-text documents. Finally, *BibSonomy* with 3.5 million and *Zotero* with 2.5 million are products that contain the lowest number of materials which confirms their reduced scope of activity.

The reason for the outstanding performance of *Mendeley* and *ResearchGate* could be the fact that their databases are not only fed directly by their users, but that both sites extract bibliographic information from secondary sources. In the case of *Mendeley*, references mainly come from PubMed and Scopus, while *ResearchGate* takes its metadata from open repositories. It is also necessary to note that the possibility of uploading a full-text document in a sharing site is much more limited than posting a reference in a reference manager or social bookmarking site, so data on *ResearchGate* and *Academia.edu* have to be even better acknowledged. For example, *ResearchGate*, with its 19 million full-text copies, is now the top supplier of full-text documents to Google Scholar, which shows the transformational power this tool has in the scholarly world (Jamali & Nabavi, 2015).

As with users, the content production rate is also an indicator of the growth of the network and points to the increasing health of the site with the addition of new documents. Annual growth rate was calculated in only four sites: *ResearchGate*, *CiteULike*, *Academia.edu* and *BibSonomy*, the remaining sites not containing historic data that would facilitate the computation. The site that experienced the highest annual growth is *ResearchGate*, with an exceptional 320 per cent. However, this was only calculated from full-text documents during the 2012–15 period, and would possibly be a much lower percentage for all documents and the full life period. Next, *Academia.edu* describes a growth of 43 per cent, followed by *BibSonomy* (27 per cent) and *CiteULike* (20 per cent). Nevertheless, if only the last five years are considered, the growth of *BibSonomy* (13 per cent) and *CiteULike* (7 per cent) is clearly reduced, which confirms again the decline of the social bookmarking sites. Overall, the results show that the services which supply most content (*Mendeley*, *ResearchGate* and *BiomedExperts*) are those that are fed from other secondary sources. It goes to show that the determination of the users is not enough to maintain an up to date and complete information system, and demonstrates that a collaborative environment is not a suitable model for creating acceptable bibliographic resources.

6.1.2.1 Disciplinary Distribution

Another important aspect of the publications referenced or deposited in social sites is the thematic distribution on each social site. As information sources, these spaces are used to obtain bibliographical information and knowing a site's disciplinary coverage helps in the choice of which platform to use to find relevant documents. Also, the thematic distribution of a social site is of interest in order to decide whether to participate or not in the site because users tend to take part in spaces where they are familiar with the content that the service offers.

Only four sites, the two reference management sites and the two sharing sites, thematically arrange their publications: *Academia.edu*, *ResearchGate*, *Mendeley* and *Zotero*. The remaining platforms have not been studied for several reasons: they do not contain any publications (*Nature Network*), they are specialized sites (*BiomedExperts*, *UniPHY*) or they do not use any classification scheme as with the social bookmarking sites (*CiteULike*,

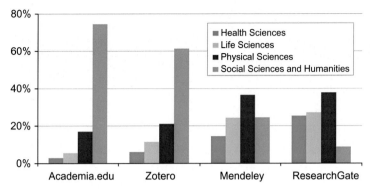

Figure 6.6 Number of publications by research area in each social site.

BibSonomy). As with profiles, publications were classified according to the Elsevier scheme. *Academia.edu* (74 per cent) and *Zotero* (61 per cent) show a clear bias toward Social Sciences and Humanities, because the presence of humanities scholars and social scientists is very high to other academic social sites (Figure 6.6). The other research areas show very low percentages, with the exception of Physical Sciences that is around 20 per cent in both sites. On the other hand, *Mendeley* and *ResearchGate* describe opposite patterns. The distribution of publications is more balanced, predominantly Physical Science with 37 per cent and 38 per cent documents and Life Sciences with 24 per cent and 27 per cent respectively. *ResearchGate* is the site that presents most biomedical content with 25 per cent of the papers, a percentage near to the proportion of physicians registered in the site. As was said in the Profiles section, *Academia.edu* and *Zotero* could be considered specialized networks because the great majority of content corresponds to Humanities and Social Sciences, while *Mendeley* and *ResearchGate* are balanced platforms with a similar thematic distribution comparable to other scientific information resources (i.e. citation indexes, scientific databases, search engines). The equilibrium in these two sites could be related to the fact that both sites take many of their publications from external sources. It is possible that this practice provides them with stability of content and therefore they are more attractive to a wider range of scholars. Otherwise, on comparing the distribution of profiles and publications, it is interesting to observe that the presence of Social Sciences and Humanities profiles in *ResearchGate* and *Mendeley* is higher than the same proportion for publications. This could indicate that this type of user produces less content than scientists from other disciplines.

6.2 NETWORKING ACTIVITY

Apart from the number of users and items that are posted to a site, an academic social site is fuelled by the different actions that the members can carry out in the platform. The number of actions and the periodicity of them, the percentage of active users involved in viewing, posting or tagging publications, and the way in which users collaborate among themselves in groups and forums are indices that measure the energy of a network. A system without activity, then, is a space destined to grind to a gradual standstill, a site where the content has become obsolete and its users have lost interest, soon to head towards disappearance. However, a very active network is an up to date and fresh space that increases its value more and more and invites new scholars to participate.

A primary indicator of activity in an academic social site is the amount of content that their members make to add to the system, because a site with a lot of posted items means that their users are very active uploading materials. The average of items posted to the platform measures the intensity of participation in adding publications, while the percentage of posters is the ratio of members that take actively part in the service.

Some sites were excluded from this analysis as it was not possible to calculate these indicators using the data extracted from the site. *Nature Network* and *Zotero* only included this information in groups and forums, which will be analysed later, while *BiomedExperts* and *UniPHY* automatically fed their databases from external sources. The most active members posting publications are on *BibSonomy*, with 77 references posted on average, followed by *ResearchGate* (35.5), *CiteULike* (25.7) and *Mendeley* (24.9) (Figure 6.7). This heightened activity in *BibSonomy* is in contrast with its

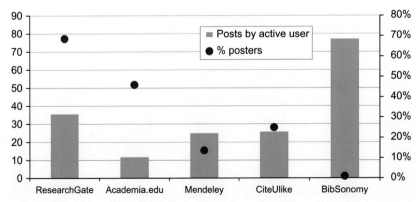

Figure 6.7 Average of posts by user and percentage of users posting in each social site.

very low degree of participation (0.97 per cent) which could be due to a very small group of active users (0.97 per cent), many of whom are creators themselves and have a frenetic rate of posting. Thus this platform survives thanks to this very active group that maintains all the activity on the site. However, these comparisons have to be taken with caution because not all posting activities involve the same effort. Document sharing sites such as *Academia.edu*, *ResearchGate* and *Mendeley*[1] only permit references or full-texts authored by the user him or herself to be uploaded, while social bookmarking sites accept any type of bibliographic reference without any limitation. *Academia.edu*, for example, only allows full-text documents authored by users themselves to be posted, which means that the average of items posted by person (11.7) is among the lowest. However, the percentage of users (46 per cent) posting material is the second highest, confirming that the network is very active uploading documents, but that the number of items that users can contribute is limited by their scientific production and the restrictions of the publishing houses. *ResearchGate* (35.5 posts by user) and *Mendeley* (24.9 posts by user) show better figures because full-texts are optional. Nevertheless, while *ResearchGate* describes the highest percentage of users including references (68.6 per cent), *Mendeley* presents the second worst participation percentage (13.7 per cent). Unlike in *Academia.edu*, this difference is due to *Mendeley* being mainly used as a reference manager and its users do not employ their profiles to boost their publications. In general, the document sharing sites *ResearchGate* and *Academia.edu* show the best participation percentages, while bookmarking sites describe low participation but a positive level of activity.

Another activity indicator is the number of followers and followings of a user. This networking functionality allows members to be updated on the activities of specific users at all times and can be used as an instrument for information searching. However, the number of followers and followings could be proxies of the degree of interaction among the social network members. Specifically, followers could be a metric that measures the interest of the online community in the activity of certain profiles, while followings might be an activity index on the information needs of a user in being updated on other colleagues' outputs.

Information on followings and followers were obtained from the two major document sharing sites, *ResearchGate* and *Academia.edu*, and both reference managers, *Mendeley* and *Zotero*. *CiteULike* implements a similar function to explore other people's libraries, but this was not quantified. Document sharing sites are the spaces that have the most active networks (Figure 6.8). *Academia.edu* is thus the site that has the most

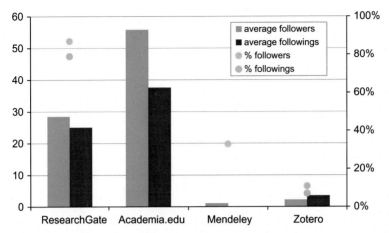

Figure 6.8 Average of followers/followings and percentage of users with followers/followings.

energized network with an average of 55.8 followers and 37.6 followings, while *ResearchGate* has 28.5 followers and 25 followings on average. This difference between *Academia.edu* and *ResearchGate* could be due to the size of the networks because *Academia.edu* has four times more users. However, *Mendeley* and *Zotero* show very low averages (<5) which confirms that this functionality is rarely used. When we consider the percentage of followers/followings, these differences are even greater, with only 33 per cent of profiles having followers in *Mendeley*, while the percentage of followers (11 per cent) and followings (7 per cent) in *Zotero* are almost irrelevant. These results confirm that this networking utility is frequently used in document sharing sites because it is the most effective way to obtain information on new contributions to the network. *Mendeley*, which also acts as a document sharing site, presents very low values because, perhaps, users do not consider this site as somewhere to exchange documents. The remaining sites provide evidence that this function makes less sense in environments where users search bibliographic references rather than authors.

6.2.1 Groups, the Collaborative Tool

Up to this point, the activity of academic social sites has been explored from an individual view, analysing how each user posts and follows other users. Now, the way in which users group together to produce some action is studied. Groups can be considered the main collaboration

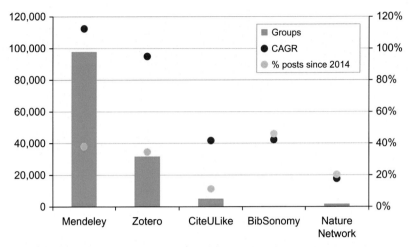

Figure 6.9 Number of groups, annual growth and percentage of items since 2014 in each social site.

instrument of an academic social site because under this instrument different users can carry out tasks together with other members. In this way, this space allows us to observe to what extent users from a social site employ the service more for collaboration activities than for individual purposes.

This instrument is not available in all the academic sites studied. The document sharing services *ResearchGate* and *Academia.edu* do not have any similar function, while *BiomedExperts* and *UniPHY* also lack of this element. Figure 6.9 shows the number of groups created in each site, in addition to the annual growth in items posted and the percentage of items posted to groups since 2014 (since 2012 in *Nature Network*). *Mendeley* is the site that has the most public groups (97,857), followed by *Zotero* (31,783) and *CiteULike* (5,085). The large number of groups in *Mendeley* – three times the number in *Zotero* – could be due to the difference between them in the number of users. It seems that reference management sites are more successful in the creation of groups than bookmarking sites. Thus the growth rate of new content in *Mendeley* (112 per cent) and *Zotero* (94 per cent) is much higher than in *CiteULike* (42 per cent) and *BibSonomy* (42 per cent), pointing out the standstill reached by social bookmarking sites and the strength of reference managers as collaborative spaces. The percentage of items posted since 2014 is a measure of group updating as the more posts are located after that period the more current are their content. Thus, *BibSonomy* (46 per cent) has the most updated

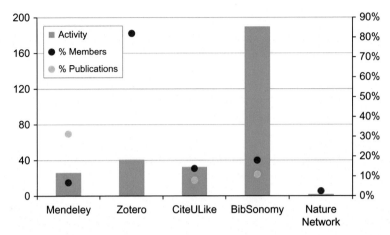

Figure 6.10 Activity, percentage of members and percentage of publications in each social site.

groups, followed by *Mendeley* (38 per cent) and *Zotero* (35 per cent). As has been seen, *BibSonomy* is supported by a small number of users that generate a huge amount of activity. This energy is also transferred to groups, as users are utilizing groups as the main networking space.

Another aspect to evaluate in groups is their activity in the context of the entire site, as a means to analysing the weight of these collaborative instruments in the entire activity of the service. Figure 6.10 shows the activity of these groups, calculated as the ratio of the number of posts in each group to the number of members affiliated to this same group. In addition, the percentage of users that decide to join to a group as well as the percentage of items posted to groups in relation to the entire site are calculated. *BibSonomy* (189.8) again shows by far the highest activity due to the reason given above − a lot of activity is being produced by a small number of users. *Zotero* (40.1) and *CiteULike* (32.6) also describe good activity rates but with five times lower activity than *BibSonomy*. In relation to the proportion of users attracted to groups, *Zotero* (82 per cent) is the platform in which most users are linked to groups, followed by *BibSonomy* (18 per cent) and *CiteULike* (14 per cent). The excessive proportion in *Zotero* could be due to the fact that most of the users are signed up to this service almost exclusively to participate in groups. However, *Mendeley* (31 per cent) is the site with the most content supplied to groups, followed by *BibSonomy* (10 per cent) and *CiteULike* (8 per cent). One reason for this could be that Mendeley has the largest bibliographic database, which helps the posting of items to groups.

In general, reference management sites are employing groups more profusely than the other platforms, creating a larger number of groups and a greater increase in their activity. This can also be seen in the weight that groups have in the entire site, with a higher percentage of publications and members involved in these collaborative tools. This has come about, firstly by the higher collaborative possibilities of the reference management sites which make possible the generation of bibliographies and the addition of references to personal libraries, and secondly by the gradual stagnation of social bookmarking sites in which activity is going down and limited to small communities such as *BibSonomy*.

6.3 CONSOLIDATION OF THE SELF-ARCHIVING PLATFORMS

The results of the comparison above have described the different performances of each social site in context with the other platforms, observing how they evolve and work in relation to their competitors. Thanks to the quantitative approach, several metrics were designed to quantify the activity, evolution, content and networking of each service, which makes it possible to equitably compare scholarly sites among and between the different types. As a result, document sharing services have demonstrated that, at the present time, they are the most successful platforms in the panorama of academic social sites. These different benchmarking analyses have provided evidence that they are the sites that attract most scholars and report better prospects for growth. Also, activity indicators have pointed out that their communities are the most energized, and the rate of following among users and the contribution of content is the highest. On the other hand, the remaining platforms show some weaknesses that confirm their obsolescence. Thus, for example, social bookmarking sites have verified that their time has passed. The size of their networks in terms of both people and content is very small and their future prospects are not favourable. The activity of these sites produces average results and even in the best cases they only survive in small, local communities such as *BibSonomy*. However, the decay of *CiteULike* is evident in every sense with a constant shrinkage in the number of posts and new affiliations. In the case of the reference management sites, *Zotero* remains just a utility for sharing bibliographies in small groups. *Mendeley* by contrast has the strength of the largest bibliographic database and an important online community which allows it to maintain the most active groups. However, the weak spot of this platform is its poor performance as a document sharing site. In this sense, *Mendeley's* users do not take advantage of their profiles, uploading very few documents and having a non–existent networking activity.

NOTE

1. In this section Mendeley is interpreted as a document sharing site. The percentage of posters and average of publications per user do not refer to the references added to the user's library, but to the publications of the users themselves posted in their profiles.

REFERENCES

Jamali, H. R., & Nabavi, M. (2015). Open access and sources of full-text articles in Google Scholar in different subject fields. *Scientometrics* Available from: <http://link.springer.com/article/10.1007/s11192-015-1642-2> 10.09.15.

Reed, R. (2001). The law of the pack. *Harvard Business Review, February*, 23–24. Available from: <https://hbr.org/2001/02/the-law-of-the-pack> 10.09.15.

CHAPTER 7

Final Remarks

This path through diverse academic platforms has made it possible to derive a general picture about their working, capacities, functionalities, purposes and performance. All these services were born in the short period 2006–8, so they are no longer young start-ups hesitant in behaviour, but they have been around long enough to display a clear view of the purposes that they want to accomplish, the model that they aim to develop and the results that they can obtain from this approach. This analytical dissection has also permitted us to observe the different types of platforms that have evolved into a consolidated model, have fallen into decline or have inevitably disappeared. In this way, this quantitative survey has brought a number of results that allow us to formulate several general conclusions regarding these web places and their future prospects.

7.1 CONTENT AS THE UNDERLYING FACTOR OF SOCIAL NETWORK DEVELOPMENT

The first conclusion is that the success or decline of a platform is intimately related to the type of content that it manages. Document sharing systems are positioned as the most successful spaces both for content generation and social networking, in addition to which this type of scholarly social networking site displays better future prospects. On the other hand, social bookmarking sites present an outdated model with a general drop in users, documents and activity that reflects the stagnation of the folksonomy as a paradigm for the creation of social networking sites. Reference management sites, considered to be a more sophisticated version of bookmarking sites, did not take off as social platforms although they remain active as a desktop application for private purposes. It is possible to claim that the achievement of a platform is strongly related to the type of services that it offers and the information or content that it manages. Thus, the sharing of full-text documents is the solution that attracts most scholars as this is the essential activity that researchers have always done in order to be up to date and connected with the most recent and

Social Network Sites for Scientists.
ISBN 978-0-08-100592-7

current advances in their fields (Vickery, 2000). On the other hand, the sharing of references is only important for bibliographic tasks and information searching which, as has been seen, only attracts the attention of students and young scholars. Content thus emerges as the key element in the working of these platforms and determines the most successful architecture. It is not surprising that designs such as Nature Network, BiomedExperts and UniPHY have disappeared, as their models did not take into account the exchange and production of content. In the case of Nature Network the networking system was basically based on forums and discussion groups, while BiomedExperts and UniPHY simply did not include any instrument for sharing information among their profiles. With regard to the social bookmarking sites (CiteULike and BibSonomy) and reference managers (Mendeley and Zotero), bibliographic reference is the main information unit that these platforms put in circulation. In these sites, users act as collaborative collectors that interchange and post bibliographic citations with the aim of creating self-organized information systems. In the case of document sharing services (Academia.edu and ResearchGate), documents are now the key materials, shared by the authors themselves through the uploading of full-text copies to their respective profiles. It could therefore be possible to think that there is an evolving change in the nature of these academic sites, in which the content has played a central role in the adaptation and transformation of these models. Thus, from a initial uncertain approach in which it was expected that users would only be put in contact through forums and groups, an active model was developed in which tagging and posting references was the force that shaped the network. This was finally finished with a framework focused on the establishment of networking ties from the exchange of the creations of the users themselves.

7.2 ACTIVITY DEFINES THE TYPOLOGY OF USERS AND SITE USAGE

The second conclusion is that participation in these platforms is diverse and influenced by the type of service and users. The definition of participation may be blurred and depends on the platform type, the activities that can be developed there and the amount of content that a user could post. Nielsen (2006) explains the 90-9-1 rule which states that 90 per cent of users do not participate in anything, 9 per cent contribute a little and 1 per cent make most of the contributions. However, this rule is not exact and the variations could be used as an indicator of activity and inequality. Nentwich and König (2014) count five types of users according to their degree of participation and suppose that those with the lowest activity are the most frequent users. In our study, if participation is considered to be the number of users that post something to the network, the empirical results show that, in the best-case scenarios, participation is 68 per cent (ResearchGate) and 46 per cent (Academia.edu), while in the worst it is 14 per cent (Mendeley) and 0.9 per cent (BibSonomy). In any case, the results show values higher than estimated by Nielsen's rule which suggests that the activity in academic social sites is higher than in other web spaces. Moreover, the percentages are very different among them and demonstrate that the participation levels are not the same across platforms, but that the type of activity that these sites develop could be the main influence on the involvement of members. Document sharing services present by far much higher activity than the other services, suggesting that the exchange of documents is a more attractive activity for users than posting references or tagging bookmarks. However, this view if participation is rather flat and only considers whether the user posts or does not post content. The analysis of these spaces has brought us to observe that the degree of participation is much more complex and that users' activity could be expressed in very different ways. Thus, different typologies of users emerge to develop different activities according their needs and the possibilities of the service. In the case of Academia.edu, this fact was clearly observed when two types of users were detected: viewers make up the majority many of whom are *independent* users that mainly follow the research activity of other users but scarcely put in content of their own. On the contrary, producers form a smaller group of highly productive researchers that post a large amount of items but they are not interested in following the activity of the network. To some extent, these different types of users arise from the different needs that they have and how they can satisfy them in the platform. In Mendeley, for example, there are four million users with poor networking rates and one of the lowest proportions of users posting content (14 per cent), joining groups (6 per cent) or following members (33 per cent). In this case, users perceive Mendeley more as a private desktop application than as a social networking place. Following this idea, it is possible that many of the passive users observed by Nielsen (2006) and Nentwich and König (2014) would correspond to members that employ these spaces as information resources wherein they explore the site looking for new and up-to-date content, instead of posting items, setting up collaboration groups or responding to questions. This leads us to bear in mind that participation in these spaces consumes a significant amount of time, which would explain why most users have just a basic presence.

7.3 DIOGENES CLUB? PRIVATE OVER PUBLIC INTERESTS

The third conclusion is that users move toward scholarly social networks more for egotistical motives than for collaborative purposes. In a world in which participation in academic social networks has been lauded as an example of the cooperative nature of Science (Calhoun, 2014; Cann, Dimitriou, & Hooley, 2011; Zaugg, West, Tateishi, & Randall, 2011), and where these spaces have been associated with the altruistic spirit of the scholarly community, it is surprising to state that these networking platforms are in the main not being used for collaborative purposes but rather for personal matters. Although we talk on social networking sites, many of these platforms allow the use of these spaces for individual purposes without the need to establish contacts or enter into collaborations with other users. In other words, it could be said that these sites are not so much a meeting room where users chat and develop activities together, but are rather personal spaces where individual actions can be taken advantage of by other members. The reason for the small fraction of 'active' users could be due to the remaining members using the network for private purposes, viewing the information that others post, witnessing the discussions that others initiate and tracking the statistics that their publications produce. Social bookmarking sites, the best examples of collaborative space, in truth, are a collection of private libraries made public in which the rest of the users can reuse the work of others. Even then, only 26 per cent of CiteULike's and 10 per cent of BibSonomy's members have posted something in their libraries. The remaining members could be using the libraries of others to be up-to-date on specific issues and/or as a specialized information resource. Seen in other way, a few users put a lot of content in a network so that the great majority can capture the most beneficial items for them. Groups, a service precisely oriented to the collaboration between users (Oh & Jeng, 2011), is the clearest example of the poor interest of this community in taking part in joint activities. Hence, the percentage of users enrolled in groups is 13.9 per cent in CiteULike and 18 per cent in BibSonomy, while the average number of posts to groups is lower than the same average to the entire network in CiteULike (18.6 in groups; 25.7 in the network).

The situation with reference management sites is not much better. Mendeley and Zotero were created as desktop applications for individual needs and their jump to the social networking environment has not been as good as expected. In their regard, the system is only able to make public the references that their users want. In Mendeley, the 'public catalogue' only contains 12 per cent of all the items posted to the service, showing that their users are not willing to share their references. This pattern is also repeated in Zotero where only 4 per cent of users' libraries are public. Nor have the networking spaces of these services taken off sufficiently either. Mendeley's network only has an average of 1 follower per user, while 14 per cent of their users have scarcely added any papers to their profiles. Zotero describes similar networking figures with 11 per cent of followers and 7 per cent of followings. These data confirm the poor networking activity of these platforms and, as in social bookmarking sites, it appears that most of their users only want to manage their own libraries and exploit the public catalogue to capture references. The use of groups is also similar to social bookmarking sites. In Mendeley, only 8 per cent of users are joined to groups and the post average in these services (16.7) is lower than in the entire network (24.9). These results do nothing but cast doubts on the utility of a social networking site in products that mainly offer one service – references management – for purely private purposes.

The situation with document sharing sites is a little different. In these spaces, the main intention is to share publications between their members, which means that the participation levels are higher. Thus, 68 per cent of ResearchGate's users and 46 per cent of Academia.edu's post some items to the platform. However, while these rates do not reveal an altruistic behaviour, they could be motivated by a conceited need to monitor the use and impact of their publications in the academic world. The range of metrics that describe the performance of papers, profiles and organizations, and the dashboards that track the usage of the users' publications, are instruments that encourage the publishing of results, but do not promote collaboration at all. According to networking metrics, these spaces are also the most active with the highest average of followers and followings. However, these activity levels could be not motivated by social or connection needs, but they might be used for searching information. Thus, as we have seen in Academia.edu, many of the users that principally follow profiles are also members who provide little content. In this sense, followers could be users that focus their activity on seeking information through the updates they receive from their followings. On the contrary, producers, who post many publications but follow few people, employ the application mainly for disseminating their output. In this way, both types of users might not be centred in collaboration activities, but they could be looking to meet their personal needs. Questions & Answers is the only collaboration tool used in this type of social networking place, which provides evidence of the limited interest that document sharing sites have in the collaboration process. This function reveals that only 1 per cent of users launch a query and just one in seven follows the replies to these queries, showing again the poor attention to participative environments in the academic community.

To summarize, academic participation in these virtual spaces is more like a kind of Diogenes Club[1] where all the members come together to do private and personal things, while freely taking advantage of the work of their colleagues. To some extent, the academic contacting network is based on a rewards system in which an elite of highly prestigious producers use these spaces to spread their productions in return for watching the impact that these materials are provoking in a huge community of young scholars and academics from developing countries who are following this production so they can be up to date in specific fields.

7.4 METRICS FOR MANAGING REPUTATION AND SOCIALIZING, NOT FOR RESEARCH IMPACT

The fourth conclusion is that social sites for scholars cannot be a substitute, at the present time, for the current scholarly reward system, not even as an alternative. The reasons for this statement include a wide variety of matters. The first is the previous need to define the sense of these indicators and their implications for the research assessment of individuals, papers and organizations. It is easy to précis the meaning of citations, publications, etc., as proxies of scholarly production and impact, but metrics such as views, readers and followers come from very different actions and the significance of these indicators for the evaluation of research is not still clear (Sugimoto, 2015). Perhaps more research studies are needed to uncover the real meaning of these metrics and see to what extent they reflect the type of impact they have and whether, in the end, this is related to academic excellence and prestige. At the moment, many studies have only found average correlations among these measurements caused, in most of the cases, by multiple and uncontrolled interactions (Li, Thelwall, & Giustini, 2012; Ortega, 2015; Thelwall & Kousha, 2014, 2015). Another limitation is that these online networking spaces are closed and their usage, networking and impact metrics are calculated on activity inside the network. This means that similar metrics such as followers/followings, views, downloads, etc., could express different results across platforms so that, for example, users with a high rate of views in one place could go unnoticed in another site. This is explained not only by the intrinsic technical differences in extracting and computing these indicators or simply by the number of users, but also by the important geographical and thematic biases that these populations present. Yet while there are sites mainly occupied by researchers from the same country (Bibsonomy, Zotero), others are unbalanced toward certain disciplines (Academia.edu) and in other cases students surpass the population (Mendeley). These biases could influence these indicators in such way that would make it almost impossible to benchmark between metrics from different services. Another problem not adequately taken into account is the length of time a user or paper is included in a social platform (Thelwall & Kousha, 2014). Networking (i.e. followers) and usage (i.e. views) indicators are also time-dependent metrics, increasing their value according to the length of time that a profile is active on a particular site and which could be different had the profile been on a different site. In other words, the metrics of one user who has been registered in a service for a length of time would be higher than if the author had recently signed up. Another important fact is that signing up to these services is voluntary and the adoption rate by this part of the research community is generally low and different across sites (Haustein et al., 2014; Mas-Bleda, Thelwall, Kousha, & Aguillo, 2014). This means that it is difficult to evaluate some authors while the global view on organizations and research disciplines could be incomplete and limited. Despite these limitations, however, these reputation metrics do offer additional information on the influence of an author and the usage of their research outputs on their online scientific network, describing a different and social dimension to the place that a researcher occupies in the scholarly community. These measurements therefore must also be appreciated but only as signs of networking, popularization and socializing.

7.5 TOWARD A SOCIETAL COMMITMENT OF THE SCIENTIST TO THE CITIZENSHIP

The fifth and last conclusion is that scholars should get involved in these spaces because of their commitment to the citizens in general and to being transparent to society. In general, one of the changes that the Web brought was that people searched for scientific information with more assiduity and interest, which entailed a higher perception of science and a closer understanding of the scholarly activity on the part of society (Ripberger, 2011). However, it also brought about more public judgement of the research activity as well as increasing the impact of scientific results on daily life (i.e. Medicine, Environmental Science, Economics, Information Technologies, etc.) (Leach, Scoones, & Wynne, 2005). For example, many of the *independent* users of Academia.edu may not be academics looking for updates to issues in which they are interested. Citizens thus have the right to demand responsibility and results from scientists, not only because the last addressee of the research outputs is society itself, but also because many of the researchers are civil servants and their research investigations are funded by public resources (Hagendijk & Irwin, 2006). In this way, researchers have a public commitment to society to which they have to answer (Molloy, 2011). Hence social networking places are ideal locations where scholars should make public their academic outputs so that society can appreciate the importance of their contributions and be sure of the efforts these professionals make (Martorell & Canet, 2013). Usage (views, downloads) and networking (followers) metrics are good indicators that fit in with the context of the popularization of science and societal impact. This transparent attitude could be an important way to justify the enormous budgets allocated to R&D, and to move the citizenship closer to academic culture. In other words, organizations and countries should promote the use of academic social sites as a way to persuade society of the importance to the country's health of funding science. Thus a society aware of the efforts of its scientists is a society that will better understand the problems and needs of the scholarly community.

NOTE

1. Diogenes Club is the name of the club co-founded by the brother of Sherlock Holmes, Mycroft Holmes. The only rule of this club was that it was not allowed to talk with other members, being an ironic view of Victorian society and the allure of social clubs.

REFERENCES

Calhoun, K. (2014). *Exploring digital libraries: Foundations, practice, prospects*. London and Chicago: Facet Publishing and ALA Neal-Schuman.
Cann, A., Dimitriou, K., & Hooley, T. (2011). *Social media: A guide for researchers*. London: Research Information Network. Available from: <http://www.rin.ac.uk/our-work/communicating-and-disseminating-research/social-media-guide-researchers> 10.09.15.

Hagendijk, R., & Irwin, A. (2006). Public deliberation and governance: Engaging with science and technology in contemporary Europe. *Minerva, 44*(2), 167–184.

Haustein, S., Peters, I., Bar-Ilan, J., Priem, J., Shema, H., & Terliesner, J. (2014). Coverage and adoption of altmetrics sources in the bibliometric community. *Scientometrics, 101*(2), 1145–1163.

Leach, M., Scoones, I., & Wynne, B. (2005). *Science and citizens: Globalization and the challenge of engagement* (vol. 2). New York: Zed Books.

Li, X., Thelwall, M., & Giustini, D. (2012). Validating online reference managers for scholarly impact measurement. *Scientometrics, 91*(2), 461–471.

Martorell, S., & Canet, F. (2013). Shared secrets: Web 2.0 and research in Social Sciences. *ESSACHESS – Journal for Communication Studies, 6*(2), 45–64.

Mas-Bleda, A., Thelwall, M., Kousha, K., & Aguillo, I. F. (2014). Do highly cited researchers successfully use the social web? *Scientometrics, 101*(1), 337–356.

Molloy, J. C. (2011). The open knowledge foundation: Open data means better science. *PLoS Biol, 9*(12), e1001195.

Nentwich, M., & König, R. (2014). Academia goes Facebook? The potential of social network sites in the scholarly realm. In S. Bartling & S. Friesike (Eds.), *Opening science* (pp. 107–124). New York, NY: Springer International.

Nielsen, J. (2006). *The 90-9-1 rule for participation inequality in social media and online communities.* Nielsen Norman Group. Available from: <http://www.nngroup.com/articles/participation-inequality/> 10.09.15.

Oh, J. S., & Jeng, W. (2011). Groups in academic social networking services – an exploration of their potential as a platform for multi-disciplinary collaboration: *2011 IEEE Third International Conference on Privacy, Security, Risk and Trust (PASSAT)*. Washington: IEEE Computer Society; 545–548.

Ortega, J. L. (2015). Relationship between altmetric and bibliometric indicators across academic social sites: The case of CSIC's members. *Journal of Informetrics, 9*(1), 39–49.

Ripberger, J. T. (2011). Capturing curiosity: Using Internet search trends to measure public attentiveness. *Policy Studies Journal, 39*(2), 239–259.

Sugimoto, C. (2015). "Attention is not impact" and other challenges for altmetrics. *Exchanges Our Ideas, Research and Discussion Blog.* Available from: <http://exchanges.wiley.com/blog/2015/06/24/attention-is-not-impact-and-other-challenges-for-altmetrics/> 10.09.15.

Thelwall, M., & Kousha, K. (2014). Academia.edu: Social network or academic network? *Journal of the Association for Information Science and Technology, 65*(4), 721–731.

Thelwall, M., & Kousha, K. (2015). ResearchGate: Disseminating, communicating, and measuring scholarship? *Journal of the Association for Information Science and Technology, 66*(5), 876–889.

Vickery, B. (2000). *Scientific communication in history.* Lanham, MD: Scarecrow Press.

Zaugg, H., West, R. E., Tateishi, I., & Randall, D. L. (2011). Mendeley: Creating communities of scholarly inquiry through research collaboration. *TechTrends, 55*(1), 32–36.

INDEX

Note: Page numbers followed by "*f*" and "*t*" refer to figures and tables, respectively.

Printed in the United States
By Bookmasters